REGULATION AND
DRUG DEVELOPMENT

Evaluative Studies

This series of studies seeks to bring about greater understanding and promote continuing review of the activities and functions of the federal government. Each study focuses on a specific program, evaluating its costs and efficiency, the extent to which it achieves its objectives, and the major alternative means—public and private—for reaching those objectives. Yale Brozen, professor of economics at the University of Chicago and an adjunct scholar of the American Enterprise Institute for Public Policy Research, is the director of the program.

REGULATION AND DRUG DEVELOPMENT

William M. Wardell
and
Louis Lasagna

American Enterprise Institute for Public Policy Research
Washington, D. C.

This study is one of a series published by the American Enterprise Institute as part of the research program of AEI's Center for Health Policy Research. A distinguished advisory committee, whose members are listed below, helps guide this program.

ISBN 0-8447-3167-6

Evaluative Studies 21, July 1975

Library of Congress Catalog Card No. 75-18947

Printed in the United States of America

CONTENTS

INTRODUCTION

In the late 1950s the Congress of the United States began holding subcommittee hearings on various matters pertaining to the pharmaceutical industry. Two of the most vigorous and sensational were those chaired by Congressman Blatnik and by Senator Kefauver. They were highly critical of the quality of drug advertising, the evidence for effectiveness of marketed pharmaceuticals, the allegedly monopolistic nature of the drug industry, and the price of medicines.

The drug industry, accustomed to respect and gratitude from physicians and the public, was suddenly confronted with hostile, sensational newspaper headlines and stories and a rising wave of angry criticism. Despite the furor, legislation almost certainly would not have ensued were it not for the thalidomide disaster. The epidemic of grossly deformed "seal babies" (practically all of whom were European) almost overnight achieved the unanimous passage of the Drug Industry Act of 1962, the so-called Kefauver-Harris amendments to the Food, Drug and Cosmetic Act of 1938. The fact that thalidomide had not been approved for U.S. marketing was somehow irrelevant, as was the fact that the new requirements in the amendments, had they been in effect, would not have prevented a thalidomide-type tragedy. The specter of drug toxicity sufficed to carry the day.

After more than a decade's experience, it now seems appropriate to examine whether the 1962 amendments did in fact constitute a turning point in the evolution of controls over the American pharmaceutical industry, what influence they have had on the development, availability and use of therapeutic drugs in this country, and what lessons can be derived.

PART ONE

Science, Government, and the Current State of Affairs

CHAPTER I

PRE-1962 PRACTICES: THE EVOLUTION OF CONTROLS OVER THERAPEUTIC DRUGS

The original stimulus for legislation in the United States was concern over food rather than drugs. To this day, realities of medical science and practice have not always been acknowledged in the legislation or in its interpretation. One consequence has been the apparently unintended penetration of legislative and regulatory influence into the practice of medicine.

Developments Prior to the Present Century

Before the twentieth century, most food and drug controls were directed against impure and adulterated foods. This concern was produced by the social pressures and limited by the technical abilities of the period. Medicines were thought to pose problems similar to foods but were of secondary importance, except to the pharmacy profession. Indeed, much of the development of the science of pharmacy in the nineteenth century was concerned with attempts to standardize and improve the quality of prescription drugs.

Nevertheless, the seeds of today's issues of safety and efficacy were there from the beginning. Safety considerations arose in relation to the therapeutic use of frankly toxic substances—for example, the use of hydrocyanic acid in the treatment of pulmonary tuberculosis. Questions of efficacy arose in two respects: adulteration of

Much of the information in this historical account is based on James G. Burrow, *American Medical Association: Voice of American Medicine* (Baltimore: The Johns Hopkins Press, 1973), and John B. Blake, ed., *Safeguarding the Public: Historical Aspects of Medicinal Drug Control* (Baltimore and London: The Johns Hopkins Press, 1970). In the latter volume, the chapters by Glenn Sonnedecker, James Burrow, Harry Dowling, James Young and David Cavers were found to be particularly useful.

active medicines with inert fillers and false claims made for the so-called patent (secret) medicines or nostrums. These early concerns about safety and efficacy foreshadowed later concerns with these same issues, although the current issues present themselves in vastly more subtle form.

Other premonitory signs of modern controversies arose in the last century. The medical profession has long resisted the intrusion of third parties into the practice of medicine, and the novel concepts of scientific therapeutics were not above suspicion. As early as 1860, Armand Trousseau disputed the assumption that therapeutics had much to learn from science: "Far from me, gentlemen, is the thought of indicting the ancillary sciences and chemistry in particular; I only condemn the exaggeration and pretensions of these sciences, their clumsy and impertinent meddling in our art." [1] As we shall see, with a slight shift of aim so that regulatory and other third-party targets replace the objects of Trousseau's original concern with academic and paraprofessional influences, these sentiments reflect the attitude of some members of the medical profession today.

The Twentieth Century: U.S. Federal Controls

A landmark in the modern control of drugs was the 1906 Pure Food and Drugs Act. Food was considered first and drugs second. Food abuses were still the primary concern of the legislators.

Harvey Washington Wiley was the most important single figure in the long struggle to secure the law. As chief chemist of the Department of Agriculture, he wrote a long series of reports extending over sixteen years and 1,400 pages, dealing exclusively with the adulteration of food. Wiley's, and the Department of Agriculture's, emphasis on food continued until at least 1912, when he resigned. More than three-quarters of the Bureau of Chemistry's first 1,000 notices of judgment, reporting terminated cases under the law up to August 1911, were in the food field.

Less than a quarter related to drugs. Of these, the majority were concerned with patent medicines. Nostrums had for some time been considered the most threatening menace in the field of drugs. In 1903, Wiley had begun to make anti-nostrum speeches and to suggest that the definition of *drug* in the pending law should be broadened to cover proprietary remedies. In that same year, a drug laboratory was set up in Wiley's bureau. Patent medicines joined catsup and whiskey as a theme for congressional debate.

The 1906 law defined *drug* broadly and governed the labelling, but not the advertising, of any substance used to affect disease. In the first contested criminal prosecution under the law, the bureau acted against the maker of a headache mixture containing acetanilid, bearing the beguiling name of Cuforhedake-Brane-Fude.

The first serious challenge to the law occurred when a Dr. Johnson, a Kansas City proprietor of a patent medicine, maintained that the law's prohibition of false and misleading statements did not apply to therapeutic claims. This view was upheld by the Supreme Court in 1911. In response, Congress hastily passed the Sherley amendment of 1912, banning those therapeutic claims in patent medicine that were both false and fraudulent. This wording left an exploitable loophole which culminated in the case of a liniment advertised for the cure of tuberculosis. The court decided in 1922 that a maker who believed his product to be effective had no intent to defraud, and hence could not be said to be acting fraudulently. The government's loss of the liniment case undermined the modest degree of control that had been achieved.

Prescription drugs also were subject to control under the 1906 law; in fact, there was no fixed legal boundary drawn by the bureau between prescription and nonprescription medications until 1951. However, prescription medications received a lower priority for two reasons: food and patent medicine abuses were the more urgent problems, and therapeutic nihilism (exemplified by Osler and perhaps justifiable at the time) reigned in the highest echelons of American medicine. To be legal under the 1906 law, all prescription drugs had to meet the standards for composition of the *United States Pharmacopoeia* or the *National Formulary*. The Bureau of Chemistry assumed the task of examining drugs in this respect.

During the Wiley years these activities of the bureau had been concerned with the quality of plant-derived drugs. In 1912, standardization of tablets and pills and inspection of manufacturing plants were initiated. The year 1923 marked an intensification of drug control work. Bioassays were instituted of potent and crude drugs of biological origin—digitalis and ergot, for example.

Thirty years of experience with the 1906 law revealed many deficiencies. In 1933, Senator Copeland introduced a bill, prepared by the Department of Agriculture, as part of President Roosevelt's New Deal promises of domestic reform. Although the Copeland bill represented a vast improvement over the original act and for the first time would have applied federal control to the cosmetic industry, it failed to inspire much enthusiasm among the traditional supporters of more effective legislation and at the same time aroused enormous opposition.

The bill was modified several times by its sponsor over the next four years in the hope of making its passage feasible. It was only after the outrage following the Elixir Sulfanilamide [*sic*] tragedy of 1937 that Congress acted—but then with astonishing alacrity. In 1938 it passed the Wheeler-Lea act, bringing under federal regulation types of advertising not encompassed by the act of 1906. In June of that same year the Food, Drug and Cosmetic Act of 1938 was signed. It extended the government's control over advertising and labelling and required new drugs to obtain approval—indicating satisfaction of safety criteria—from the Food and Drug Administration (FDA) before being allowed in interstate commerce.

Until the Elixir Sulfanilamide episode, drug control had seemed essentially a problem of protecting the public against quacks, closing the Sherley amendment loophole requiring proof of fraudulent intent with regard to misbranding, and prohibiting the sale of dangerous drugs. Thitherto, the main object of regulatory controls had been the quality of the drug product and its labelling, although matters of safety had been broadly encompassed by the 1906 law, which had originally provided against the sale of drugs that were "dangerous to health when used [as labelled]. . . ."

Until the advent of sulfanilamide, which heralded the pharmaceutical revolution, new drugs had posed few problems because there were few of them. The Elixir Sulfanilamide disaster brought to light the specific dangers associated with new drugs and the need to test them for safety. This incident stimulated the erecting of administrative procedures for the premarketing clearance of new drugs, provisions that were among the most important of the new act.

Control over new drugs in the 1938 act was viewed not so much as a means of equipping the government to cope with a rising tide of new and hazardous drugs, but rather as a means of preventing the marketing of untested, potentially harmful drugs not generally recognized as safe by experts. For the first five years after the passage of the 1938 act, the new regulations were seen as a barrier to another Elixir Sulfanilamide tragedy. Nevertheless, at that point, and indeed until 1963, no government control over investigational plans was exerted prior to the submission of a new drug application. Manufacturers themselves learned from the Elixir Sulfanilamide experience the liability losses that could be suffered from the marketing of such drugs and instituted premarketing safety tests to avoid a repetition of this experience.

Control of prescription drugs. An obscure proviso of the 1938 act was destined to be the starting point for some of the most potent controls the FDA now exercises in the drug field. This was the power to exempt drugs, by regulation, from the requirement in

Section 502 that their labelling give adequate directions for use. The chief consequence of this exempting power was the emergence of the prescription drug as an object of special controls. The exempting regulation required that prescription drugs carry only the legend "Caution—to be used only by or on the prescription of a physician."

In 1951, the Humphrey-Durham amendment sought to define prescription drugs. That act classed drugs into three categories: (1) those labelled "Warning: May be habit forming," (2) those considered unsafe unless ádministered by a licensed physician, and (3) those new drugs limited by the terms of a Section 505 new drug application (NDA) to prescription by a licensed physician.

During the debate on this act, the question arose of whether the administrator of the Federal Security Agency (FSA), of which the FDA at that time formed a part, should be able to designate drugs for category (2) on certain criteria, one of which should be a finding that the drug is "ineffective" for use without diagnosis by, or supervision of, a licensed practitioner. The Congress concluded that it would be unwise to give this power solely to the FSA head, and that there should be a judicial hearing available as a check. The FSA head challenged this, saying that it gave the federal courts legislative authority beyond their constitutional power. This foreshadows the judicial flavor that has come to characterize therapeutic decisions in the U.S. over the past decade. The effectiveness issue is also one which increased in importance as time progressed. The reaction at the time of the American Medical Association (AMA) to this issue is described later.

Concern with problems of communication grew after passage of the 1938 amendments. A major defect of the generally strong 1938 law was found to be its lack of adequate control over advertising. In 1944, regulations were promulgated as to ways in which information on prescription drugs should be made available. The current regulations require that "labelling on or within the package from which the drug is to be dispensed" bear adequate information for its use. This is the legal explanation of the package insert. The content of an approved package insert represents a baseline from which, since 1962, the FDA has been able to measure and proceed against deviations in advertising.

Role of the Professions of Medicine and Pharmacy

Legislation and regulation do not spring spontaneously from government, and the field of therapeutic drugs affords no exception. The medical profession, working principally through the American Medical Association, was a powerful force in achieving the passage of strong legislation, particularly in the early part of the century. Even before the involvement of professional medicine, however, the profession of pharmacy played a key role in the earliest attempts at voluntary regulation and in instituting federal controls. The Philadelphia College of Pharmacy, the nation's first (founded in 1821), was greatly concerned from its beginning about "spurious and inert medicines." Concern with the control of drug quality was written into the college's constitution, whose writers viewed with alarm the varying methods in use for preparing the same drug, the availability of differing strengths of given drugs under the same name, and the difficulty of detecting adulterations, all of which they declared "offer great incitements to cupidity and open a wide door to abuses." The college's constitution provided for expulsion of any member "guilty of adulterating or sophisticating any articles of medicine or drugs, or of knowingly vending articles of that character." Supervision and maintenance of standards was one of the objects of the college. In the America of the 1820s, this supervision implied group self-discipline rather than government intervention. The New York College of Pharmacy, founded eight years later, had similar concerns.

The founding of the American Pharmaceutical Association in 1852 was a professional reaction against the emasculation of the first national law designed to control the quality of drug imports. It is clear that the earliest concerns with efficacy were pharmaceutical ones, related to adulteration and to the substitution of inert ingredients for active drugs, and that voluntary self-regulation by the pharmaceutical profession was one of the earliest effective control measures exerted over drugs.

Compulsory measures also existed. Legislation on licensing and drug adulteration was adopted by at least fourteen states before 1865. At the federal level, one of the most important relevant actions of the nineteenth century had been the passage, under pressure from the New York College of Pharmacy, of the national drug import law of 1848. However, neither the state nor federal laws of this period were effective, because of both technical and legal inadequacies.

Formularies played an important part in the specification of drug standards. They were spontaneous products of the medical and pharmacy professions. The first *United States Pharmacopoeia* was the result of a national convention held in 1820 representing all the state medical societies, colleges of physicians and surgeons, and medical schools then existing in the United States. The first edition was published in the same year.[2] By the 1842 edition, colleges of pharmacy had formally joined the endeavor. Unlike the *Pharmacopoeia,* the *National Formulary of Unofficinal [sic] Preparations* (first edition, 1888) from the beginning was prepared principally by pharmacists and published under the authority of their national professional society.

In 1881, a New Jersey law termed a drug *adulterated* if it deviated from the standards laid down in the *U.S. Pharmacopoeia*. Other states soon followed this example. The 1906 federal law gave the *Pharmacopoeia* and the *National Formulary* equal recognition as criteria for drug specifications.

A deeper involvement of the medical profession in the control of drugs began in 1900 when the AMA embarked on a program to expose the evils of nostrums. The AMA did not initiate this struggle; that honor belongs to such organizations as the Women's Christian Temperance Union and the National Temperance Society, which, along with other bodies, had formed the National Pure Food and Drug Congress in 1898. When the U.S. Congress failed to extend federal control over the manufacture of food and drugs at the close of the nineteenth centry, the AMA embarked on a program of its own to expose the nostrum evil, beginning in 1900 with a series of articles in its journal exposing the patent remedy business, as well as deficiencies in medical and surgical equipment.

In 1902, the AMA joined with the American Pharmaceutical Association to establish a committee to study such problems as drug efficacy and adulteration. This committee proposed in 1903 a "National Bureau of Medicines and Foods" which would certify the "identity, purity, quality and strength" of pharmaceutical preparations that it accepted. The committee believed that these functions were properly those of the federal government, but added that all efforts to secure federal control had failed. The expense of this bureau was to be borne by the firms dealing with it, not by the AMA. However, in 1904, the proposal was rejected by the AMA's House of Delegates.

In 1905, the House of Delegates closed the pages of the *Journal* to all nostrum advertisements. More important, it created the AMA's Council on Pharmacy and Chemistry, whose functions came to embrace the examination of both ethical and patent medicines. The reference committee chairman told the assembly that the creation of the council would be "the most important and effective measure ever undertaken by this association to rid the profession of the abuse of the nostrum evil." The first edition of *New and Non-official Remedies* was published in 1907.

These moves had the blessing of James Wilson, the U.S. secretary of agriculture, and his associates Harvey Wiley and L. F. Kebler, who pledged support and agreed to serve on the council. In this respect, the AMA was clearly the pioneer in realms now taken for granted as the preserve of government.

From 1904 to 1906, the AMA engaged in a long battle to secure passage of the Pure Food and Drugs Act, and regarded its eventual passage as a great victory in the struggle to safeguard the health of the public. A week after the President signed the bills, the *Journal* referred to passage of the measure as "too good to be true. . . . We must confess to a feeling of grateful surprise that the measure is as strong as it is."

In retrospect, it is ironic to note the AMA's pleasure that the new law provided for no appeal procedure. In the months preceding the bill's passage, the *Journal*'s editor had informed Wiley of his fear that, if the manufacturers succeeded in writing into the final measure provision for a "board of experts" to which decisions of government officials could be appealed, the measure would be vitiated. Not all the AMA's policy makers agreed with this approach, however. The *Journal*'s attack on the committee of experts deeply offended Victor C. Vaughan, dean of the University of Michigan School of Medicine and a member of the AMA's House of Delegates and Council on Medical Education, who had recommended inclusion of provision for such a committee. The conflict over this issue broke into the *Journal* and temporarily reduced the effectiveness of the crusade.

The AMA continued to campaign for strengthening the act and for its enforcement. When Wiley's judgment on sodium benzoate as a preservative failed to be supported by a presidentially appointed referee board of consulting scientific experts, the *Journal* defended Wiley's conservatism on the ground that "if he erred, he did so in the interests of the public's health instead of to the benefit of the dishonest manufacturer's pocketbook." This argument has a familiar ring today, although it is not the current position of the AMA but rather that of consumer advocates.

The *Journal* was particularly incensed by the Supreme Court's failure to consider therapeutic claims as part of the labelling of a drug. Within a month after the Court's decision on the Johnson case in 1911, the AMA adopted a resolution that soon led to the Sherley amendment of 1912, and four years later the AMA praised the Supreme Court when it upheld the constitutionality of that amendment.

In the subsequent decade, the AMA gradually became disenchanted by the weaknesses revealed in the act. The legislation did not apply to intrastate matters. The Sherley amendment's control over therapeutic claims on labels was thwarted by false advertising, over which the law had no control, and by the difficulty of proving fraudulent intent. Full disclosure was not required for labelling. The AMA considered that the attempts of the government to regulate the proprietary and patent medicine business had brought the public only limited protection.

By contrast, the AMA's Council on Pharmacy and Chemistry was strikingly successful, for several reasons. Some of the nation's leading experts were on it; the AMA staff was militantly behind its programs; and institution of the Seal of Acceptance procedure, which set out standards of identification, toxicity, efficacy, and truthfulness that a drug had to meet to be acceptable for advertisement in the association's journals, had improved advertising claims.

Gradually, the outright quacks and the fringe operators were forced out of the *Journal*'s advertising columns and sometimes out of business too. The leading companies swung round to a conformity which, though grudging, resulted in better quality products and more realistic claims for them. In 1910, the editor of the *Journal* had complained that "two directly related interests—the so-called ethical proprietary business and the 'patent medicine' business—by fair means and foul have done their best to discredit and injure the Association." In contrast, in 1946, the board of trustees could rejoice that "the Council's office has been swamped with presentations of products from firms who are now striving to bring their policies into conformance with Council principles."

In 1955, the council dropped its Seal of Acceptance program. The reasons for this change of policy were complex and have been described by the AMA itself and by the Kefauver committee, the two accounts being at variance. Senator Kefauver charged that the AMA had done this to sell more advertising. The true answer probably includes the enormous increase in the work of the program, changes of personnel and loss of the militant spirit within the AMA, and the need for substantial amounts of money to run the program. An increase in advertising revenue certainly occurred once the Seal of Acceptance was dropped; but advertising income had been rising before that point also.

The other major shift in AMA policy has been in its attitude towards government regulation of drugs. It had campaigned vigorously for the first food and drug law of 1906. During the next three decades, relationships between the AMA and the federal agencies regulating drugs remained close. The AMA and the Bureau of Chemistry of the Department of Agriculture advanced toward a common goal and kept each other informed of proposed or desired legislation, lobbying for it side by side. Wiley spoke and the *Journal* editorialized against the same quack remedies. The Department of Agriculture analyzed dubious drugs for the AMA, and the AMA obtained consultants for the Bureau of Chemistry. When it became obvious that a new law was needed, the AMA rallied to the support of friends of food and drug legislation. It wanted stronger bills than those presented in Congress and complained about weak ones. When the 1938 bill was finally passed, the AMA was disappointed that it was not stronger. It complained because the Department of Agriculture was given no control over the advertising of drugs to physicians.

For some time after 1938, the Council on Pharmacy and Chemistry continued to cooperate closely with the Department of Agriculture's successor in drug matters, the federal Food and Drug Administration. At least two secretaries of the council were recruited from the FDA during the 1940s and the staffs of the two organizations collaborated in 1944 on an article explaining how drugs should be tested. As recently as 1953, the AMA apparently approved of stronger government regulation. It proposed a bill, eventually passed, authorizing the FDA to inspect pharmaceutical laboratories without first obtaining permission from the proprietor.

Six years later there was a vast change; the AMA evidently believed regulatory laws had reached a satisfactory state. When, in 1959, Senator Kefauver began his hearings on the prices of drugs and the practices of the drug industry, the AMA lined up against the proposals for a change in the laws. The crucial provision that a drug manufacturer had to prove his claims of efficacy before he could market a drug drew fire from the AMA because "a drug's efficacy varies from patient to patient. . . . Hence any judgement concerning this factor can only be made by the individual physician who is using the drug to treat an individual patient." This was at variance with a statement approved by the board of trustees in 1954 which said that "the average physician has neither the time nor the facilities to experiment with new drugs in order to determine their proper indications for use." The AMA also opposed that portion of the proposed law which required the secretary of health, education and welfare to make determinations of what was, in effect, the relative efficacy of structurally related drugs.

A probable further factor in cooling relations between the AMA and the government was the AMA's battle against compulsory health insurance. Thus, in the early years of drug regulation, the AMA was a radical organization, probing areas of public concern far ahead of governmental action in this area. It explored new issues that were eventually incorporated in the acts of 1906, 1912, 1938, and 1962. The effectiveness of the Council on Pharmacy and Chemistry paved the way for the Food, Drug and Cosmetic Act of 1938. Likewise, the council's insistence upon valid evidence of a drug's efficacy promoted

14

such evaluations and helped improve the methodology so that, when the council dropped its Seal of Acceptance program, the federal government essentially adopted it in a more comprehensive form with the Kefauver-Harris amendments of 1962.

The AMA has clearly changed direction. Up to the 1950s, it encouraged and supported the federal government in the regulation of drugs. Since then, it has been increasingly critical, particularly of over-regulation. In this respect, it is becoming an ombudsman rather than a pilot. The AMA has also turned its attention from regulatory to educational and other efforts. In 1953, it formed a committee on blood dyscrasias, organized by Dr. Maxwell Wintrobe, that was later broadened to include all adverse drug reactions. This committee's registry, to which physicians in private practice and in hospitals could report adverse reactions, provided data for a series of articles on adverse drug reactions. In 1955, an expanded program for gathering, evaluating, and disseminating information about drugs was announced. Despite its deficiencies and its subsequent demise, the program was a primary and important step toward more exact systems of reporting.

This is a convenient point to bring up to date the story of the AMA's views on the 1962 extension of the regulation of drugs by government. The new attitude culminated at the 1973 meeting of the AMA. Six draft resolutions, from three state delegations and a specialty section, were introduced censuring the Food and Drug Administration for interfering in the practice of medicine or for not consulting with physicians specifically about drug matters. Two of the resolutions pertained primarily to the effect of the FDA on new drug development. Three of them dealt with the effects of the FDA on the availability of drug products. One alleged interference with the practice of medicine because of the agency's interpretation of the legal power of official package inserts and other labelling materials. The California state delegation proposed that the AMA seek the repeal of the 1962 Kefauver-Harris amendments and the transfer of the administration of drug matters to nongovernmental organizations such as the National Academy of Sciences.[3] The resolutions finally adopted were much watered down from the radical tone of the drafts. Nevertheless, they reflected the profession's continuing and growing concern with the incursion of government into the therapeutic relationship of physicians to their patients, and with the question of the proper and desirable scope of authority for a drug regulatory agency.

The most recent development was in June 1974, when the AMA's House of Delegates actually voted to exert all efforts to amend or repeat the Kefauver-Harris amendments, one of the arguments being that new drugs were being prevented from reaching the market.

The Climate of the 1962 Amendments

What, in fact, were the specific drug-development practices prior to 1962 to which objection was raised? To begin with, the selection of drugs for clinical trial was completely dependent on the scientific expertise and ethical conscience of sponsoring firms and clinical investigators. In the absence of legal mechanisms for regulation of clinical drug research prior to marketing, the industry was free to try a new chemical on the basis of whatever pharmacologic and toxicologic data seemed sufficient to justify such trial. Some drugs received extensive preclinical workup; others—especially if they were close congeners of drugs already demonstrated to have clinical utility and acceptable side effects—occasionally underwent the skimpiest of testing in animals. Companies varied considerably in their philosophy and practice with respect to animal experimentation. Extensive toxicity testing was not likely to be demanded by most physicians approached to perform the earliest clinical studies, so that the accumulation of such data could be postponed until after a drug was shown to have clinical utility.

Human trials were often, by today's standards, poor in design, execution, or both. In part, this reflected the state of the art at that time. Whether the legal position of the Food and Drug Administration contributed to the difficulties is a matter of dispute. The FDA was empowered, by the 1938 act, to concern itself with the safety of a product, but not specifically with its efficacy. Since no drug is absolutely safe, decisions about marketing did, in practice, take into account the use to which the drug would be put and hence its efficacy; but in theory the law's language permitted the FDA to approve a drug that was ineffective but safe.

In fact the FDA probably did not have to dissociate efficacy from safety. It has been stated by Kleinfeld that the FDA was legally able to consider efficacy even under the old 1938 act, and did so, at least on occasion.[4] The agency certainly had the premarketing mechanism of disallowing extravagant claims proposed for the package insert or "statement of directions."

Nevertheless, the FDA did not enter the picture until a manufacturer sought approval for marketing; up to this point, the responsibility for judicious decisions as to how much and what research was done with a new drug lay with the drug's sponsor and the clinicians who administered the compound to patients. Decisions as to what toxic reactions in the manufacturer's files needed to be furnished to the FDA after marketing were also the responsibility of the drug firm.

Summary and Conclusions

Legislative and regulatory controls over drugs have evolved parallel to, although somewhat behind, developments in medical and pharmaceutical sciences over the past century. Originating with the concern for detecting adulteration of foods and then drugs, progressing to the need to suppress erroneous and outrageous claims for nostrums, panaceas, and patent medicines and then to outlaw secret medicines, controls have moved from purity to safety and then more recently to concern with the efficacy of drugs and with their manner of use.

The mechanisms by which such regulation has been exerted are control over labelling (a clear heritage from the mechanism of control over the purity and content of foodstuffs), over the ability of a company to ship a drug in interstate commerce, over advertising, over investigational plans, and over the uses for which a drug is said to be approved.

Compared with the situation in previous centuries, these more recent developments in regulation are on the whole encouraging achievements, especially since many of the early steps were taken in the face of violent opposition from unscrupulous manufacturers. On the other hand, one should beware of paying excessive homage to these legal battles simply because they have been hard-fought and hard-won.

In the remainder of this volume, we will examine features of the present situation. Considering the large time lag that there has been between the need for legislation and the legislation itself, and considering the fact that some of the methods of enforcement are indirect and enter into territory not originally envisaged by the legislators, are the current laws optimal for the complex realities of modern therapeutic practice? Are by-products of the control of food adulteration and the encouragement of drug uniformity appropriate weapons for the task for which they are now being used, namely, the regulation of drug development and the practice of medicine in an attempt to ensure optimal benefit for the community? To what extent is it desirable to regulate the practice of medicine as distinct from the quality of therapeutic tools? A fundamental question is whether modern drugs and their use in the practice of medicine are most aptly controlled by regulations grounded in a philosophy evolved in a past era over concern for other substances and other problems. These are the issues which we will examine.

CHAPTER II

POST-1962 GUIDELINES AND PRACTICES

After the Kefauver-Harris amendments, drug development had to conform to a new set of guidelines. The FDA assumed a more important role in the process, especially since the issuance of regulations to implement legislation permitted considerable latitude for interpretation of the statute. While preliminary publication of regulations in the *Federal Register* does allow for criticism prior to their adoption, the *Register* is not normally perused by most of the scientific community. Therefore, serious objections by members of the academic community and the medical profession are seldom filed. Nor is the power of the FDA limited to that spelled out in law or regulations. FDA officials have opportunity, in their individual interactions with drug sponsors, to exercise qualitative or quantitative judgments that may profoundly affect the process of drug development, or to imply retaliatory action in regard to present or future drug filings to obtain industrial compliance on contested issues.

Preclinical Toxicity Testing

One of the major changes since 1962 has been in the area of preclinical toxicity testing. The sponsor of a new drug now has to submit a "Notice of Claimed Investigational Exemption for a New Drug," or Form FD 1571, to the FDA prior to human testing. The investigational new drug (IND) form is actually required to permit the interstate shipment of new drugs for clinical studies. This fact, coupled with the laying down of fairly specific guidelines by FDA experts in animal toxicology,[1] has to a large degree eliminated the giving of new drugs to man after skimpy animal testing. There have been very few instances of harm to patients resulting directly from inadequate preclinical testing of investigational drugs since the 1962 amendments. However, since there were in fact few instances *before* 1962, perhaps we need to reassess our current philosophy in regard to toxicity testing.

In contrast to the more or less general satisfaction with routine animal toxicology requirements, there is considerable controversy with respect to teratogenic, carcinogenic, and mutagenic assessments. The thalidomide story focused attention on the possibility of harm to the fetus as the result of maternal ingestion of drugs. The desire to prevent such fetal harm has, sad to say, not been matched by a concomitant development of the knowledge and techniques which would allow the goal to be achieved. As a result, exhaustive tests to measure the effect of drugs on reproduction and fetal development have been introduced, but have inspired limited enthusiasm and confidence on the part of the FDA and industrial and academic toxicologists. The data thus far obtained in monkeys are perhaps more encouraging,[2] but primate reproductive physiology poses new problems: gestation is long, multiple births are infrequent, and the supply of animals is limited.

It has long been known that many drugs, given in sufficient dosage and at appropriate time, can induce fetal damage. The extensive list includes such widely used compounds as salicylates, corticosteroids, and insulin. If a new drug demonstrates teratogenicity in any animal species, it is unlikely to be cleared for human use. If a drug is free of such effect, however, it is not assumed to be safe for consumption by women of childbearing age, since it is then said "not to have been shown to be safe" in such patients. The drug cannot be said to be safe for use by pregnant women until it has been taken by them without harm, but there is reluctance to give them the drug until it has been shown to be safe. As a result, clinical investigators often defer or avoid studies of new drugs in women of childbearing age. Manufacturers are deterred from advertising the use of such drugs in pregnancy, and doctors are liable to malpractice suits for prescribing them to pregnant women. On the surface, this might seem a generally desirable situation, since it discourages the taking of unnecessary drugs during the period of fetal development. On the other hand, we have no idea about the relative risks to the fetus of fever from untreated viral malaise in the mother and of drugs that might relieve such fever—to say nothing of the risk-benefit ratios for more serious maternal afflictions.

A similar situation exists in pediatric drug usage, with the result that most new drugs have to carry specific warnings designed to deter their use in children. Pediatricians have deplored the fact that, with respect to new drug advances, children have thus become "therapeutic orphans."

The risk of carcinogenicity deserves assessment, but there is again disagreement as to what reliance may be placed on animal testing.[3] A fundamental difference exists between the philosophical approach to ordinary toxicity testing and that to tests for teratogenicity and carcinogenicity. The former presents a scientifically logical and researchable problem; one *expects* toxic effects from an active drug when it is given in high enough dosage, and the purpose of testing is to delineate the *nature* of the toxicity and the *amount* of drug required to produce damage. These data can then be correlated with the desirable effects of the drug and the dose level at which the latter occur. One is then left with a value judgment: Is there enough leeway between therapeutic and toxic dose range, given the anticipated importance of the desirable effects, to warrant human trial?

Contrast this with the more specialized tests for teratogenicity and carcinogenicity, where many seem to be looking for an all-or-none response. The goal seems to be proof of absolute freedom from fetal damage or cancer induction. Can any drug be proven to be 100 percent safe at any dose level? Can one prove that no risk exists? Such a goal is unattainable; we should be content with suggesting that harm seems unlikely to occur under ordinary usage.

Mutagenicity testing is in an equally parlous state. A variety of subhuman tests is available, but they do not correlate well with each other, and no one is clear as to their biological meaning.

Drug metabolism has assumed greater importance as an aid to the interpretation of preclinical and clinical studies and to their design.[4] Certain applications of such data are clear and unequivocally useful, as for instance the measurement of blood or urine levels of orally administered drugs to estimate the speed and degree of absorption, metabolism, and excretion. For some drugs, individual differences in handling the chemicals seem to have important implications for their effective use. But other hopes have proved premature and doomed to disappointment, such as finding "a species like man" so that one could extrapolate from animals to humans with greater certainty. In real life, it is common to find that a drug is metabolized differently by each species, just as there may be remarkable intraspecies variation. The routine performance of metabolic studies has increased the cost and time required for new drug development; how much such studies have facilitated early testing, helped to pinpoint dosage or dosage schedules, or safeguarded patients from toxicity is a moot point.

21

Filing the IND Form

For several years after the Kefauver-Harris amendments became effective, the filing of an IND form was tantamount to permission to begin human trials. As previously discussed, irregularities in pre-clinical toxicity testing seem to have been largely eliminated for a variety of reasons, including the very need to file an IND form prior to clinical testing. There is no evidence that actual scrutiny of such toxicity data occurred with celerity and regularity on filing; limitations in FDA personnel probably precluded such a step. Comments on preclinical toxicity began to be forwarded to manufacturers late in 1970, suggesting that prompt review did not generally occur before that time. It is apparently rare for trials by industrial sponsors to be stopped on the basis of inadequacies in toxicity tests, clinical protocols, or the choice of investigators.

In the *Federal Register* of June 12, 1970, the FDA requested that a period of thirty days elapse between acknowledgment of receipt of an IND form by the FDA and the start of human testing. If the purpose of filing the form is to permit the regulatory agency to review what has been done in animals and what is planned for humans, time should obviously be allowed for perusal of the documents by the FDA staff, and the request makes sense from that standpoint.

How did the previous system, that is, no formal waiting period, work? In the *FDA Papers* for September 1969, two agency officials reviewed the experience of the post-Kefauver years.[5] Of 6,903 IND notices received by the end of fiscal 1969, 2,780 investigations were discontinued by the sponsor, most frequently because of "completing of studies, lack of commercial interest, and apparent lack of efficacy." Only 261 were terminated by the FDA, the great majority of these (188) in 1966, when the FDA staff was bolstered by the temporary assignment of a group of United States Public Health Service medical officers and pharmacists. Most of these discontinued investigations had been sponsored by individual physicians.

In the three years after September 1966, 219 IND notices were rejected on receipt. (This figure and that for terminations are presumably mutually exclusive.) The reasons for such rejection are not clearly identified in the report, but were apparently related to one or more of the following areas of supplied information: toxicology and pharmacology, chemistry and manufacturing controls, and clinical protocol. On eighteen occasions the sponsor failed to sign the form!

Why the change in regulation to introduce a waiting period after almost four years of presumably satisfactory functioning? If the new approach was proposed to provide time for scrutiny, is the thirty-day period realistic? Since the British have in recent years required approval prior to clinical trial, an analysis of their experience might be instructive.

The following data were provided on request by Pfizer, Inc.: An analysis of clinical trial submissions indicates that between 1965 and 1971, sixteen submissions on basic new agents were filed in the United Kingdom by this firm. The minimum clearance time for approval to begin clinical testing was two months and the maximum clearance time five months, the mean being three months. Half of these submissions raised queries on the part of the approving committee, as a result of which two were delayed, one by outright rejection because of an unsatisfactory submission (which was resolved by a new submission that in turn received approval within three months), and a second submission for which the committee required additional data about the identity of the drug. This occasioned a delay of approximately two months.

Data were also available concerning Pfizer submissions to extend clinical trials, to provide for new indications for a previously approved drug or to extend the range of dosage in excess of that originally approved. There were twenty-three such submissions during the period in question, with a minimum clearance time of four days and a maximum of three months. The median clearance time was approximately six weeks. Six of these submissions elicited queries from the committee, none of which produced delays.

There are problems in extrapolating from the British experience to the American scene. The committee approach utilized in Britain has not been that pursued by our FDA, and important differences exist in philosophy, quality and number of personnel, and number of submissions. Following the implementation in 1971 of the British Medicines Act, the time required to obtain a Clinical Trial Certificate first increased and subsequently fluctuated as the industry complained about what it perceived to be bureaucratic delays. A major difference between the two countries is that, in Britain, control is exerted only over the use of new drugs in *patients*. Prior to that point, drugs can, unlike in the United States, be tested in healthy volunteers without regulatory control.

If any conclusions are warranted from these analyses, the following seem reasonable. If every submission of a completely new IND notice is to be realistically scrutinized, this may require, on the average, two to three months for clearance rather than the thirty days requested by the FDA. For minor modifications in regard to previously approved drugs, a waiting period of thirty days is probably ample. An alternative approach would be to institute a selective sampling technique giving special attention to submissions that might have problems, so that these could be identified and resolved within the thirty-day period.

Seeking New Drug Application Approval

The new drug application (NDA) is not a recent phenomenon. Such applications have been required since 1938, although it is true that substantial evidence for efficacy, as well as safety, must now be supplied before a drug can be marketed.

The Kefauver-Harris amendments of 1962 eliminated the automatic approval of an NDA by the FDA in the event that the FDA failed to respond within a period of sixty days. At present, the FDA has six months to review an application. However, it is alleged that not infrequently the sponsor has often failed to receive useful feedback from the monitor until the 180 days are almost over and is then told that the NDA is defective in some regard, whereupon the process begins again. Or, it is said, at this point the FDA then requests a further delay, almost invariably given by the reluctant sponsor, which may last for months or years. The FDA used to provide status reports, quarterly during the first 180 days an NDA was under review and monthly thereafter until final disposition, but these constituted merely notification of the dates of assignment and staging without any comments on the factual content of the application.

FDA officers, on the other hand, have remarked on the poor quality of drug submissions with regard to protocol planning and execution and presentation of data.

An interesting analysis has been made of delays in NDA approvals simply on the basis of deficiencies in the chemical sections of these submissions. This survey of twenty-six Pharmaceutical Manufacturers Association (PMA) member companies indicated that sponsors could avoid a certain amount of trouble by more attention to the preparation of their filings of manufacturing and quality-control data. While a significant number of the rejections characterized by the FDA as incomplete were attributed by the PMA to "unreasonableness or inconsistency on the part of FDA reviewers" or "inadequate communication between FDA and sponsors," others were apparently caused by the submission of inadequate data.[6]

On the other hand, an analysis of six Pfizer products submitted for approval since 1965 illustrates an interesting pattern. In each case, medical review was always completed by the time other aspects of technical review were finished. The medical and technical reviews were often completed simultaneously, although in two cases it took almost two months longer for technical review. But after these reviews were completed there was then a lapse of two to twelve months before "administrative review" could be achieved. This is one place that significant delay seems to occur, and one wonders what can justify a further hiatus of one year, after expert review within the agency has approved of the fundamental aspects of the filing. The answer seems at least partly to be that, prior to 1972, the FDA statisticians were not involved in assessing the evidence until the point of administrative review had been reached. Lest the Pfizer experience be considered atypical, it may be pointed out that in the survey of twenty-six firms referred to previously, there was widespread concern over a mean of six months' time for administrative approval after completion of the technical review.

CHAPTER III

THE NATURE OF EVIDENCE

On September 19, 1969, the FDA published regulations in the *Federal Register* that defined for the first time how the agency planned to interpret the phrase "adequate and well-controlled investigations, including clinical investigations" that might elicit the "substantial evidence" of efficacy required under the 1962 Kefauver-Harris amendments. This was a new and profoundly significant turn in the history of drug assessment and therapeutics. On receipt of detailed criticism of the regulations, the FDA responded with a new set dated May 8, 1970. These contained significant improvements over the September 19 rules. (The relevant portions of the 1962 law and the 1970 regulations are reproduced in the Appendix to this volume.)

An admirable analysis of the two sets of regulations has been provided by Anello.[1] The author limits himself, to be sure, to criticisms leveled at the scientific flexibility of the stated principles and their appropriateness as a basis for well-controlled trials; he does not concern himself with such questions as hearings to settle disputes between sponsor and the FDA or the retroactive application of the regulations' principles to pre-1962 drugs.

An interesting inconsistency in the application of such principles to the evaluation of data occurs among both academic drug critics and FDA personnel. Commissioner Edwards's *Federal Register* statement of May 8, 1970, for instance, states that:

> Congress has provided that drugs introduced before 1962 shall meet the same standards of proof of effectiveness by substantial evidence as are applicable to newly developed drugs. A different and lesser standard of effectiveness is impermissible legally and would not serve the interest of patient care. Clinical experience with these drugs can and

should be considered in evaluating claims of effectiveness, but experience derived from isolated case reports, from random observations, or from clinical reports without details which permit scientific evaluation, or reports of clinical experience derived under circumstances that fall below the standards of appropriate clinical trials are of little or no value. Well documented clinical experience in an uncontrolled or partially controlled situation may be of value in contributing information as to the drug's safety, side effects, contraindications, warnings and precautionary needs. It can as well be considered as corroborative evidence, along with data derived from adequate and well-controlled clinical investigations, to support claims of effectiveness. But it cannot alone rise to the level of adequate and well-controlled clinical investigations, even when done by an experienced investigator or reported by a number of investigators who had conducted inadequately controlled clinical trials. It is not the Agency's intention to require new trials of drugs in accordance with the criteria for claims evaluated by the NAS-NRC [the National Academy of Sciences and National Research Council reviewed drugs approved between 1938 and 1962] as effective, except when the Agency has reason to draw into question any such claims at a later date based upon new information or a new evaluation.[2]

It should be noticed that the last sentence contradicts the rest of the paragraph. It is inconceivable that the National Academy of Sciences and National Research Council experts referred to (most were members of neither the academy nor the council) were able to find data of the sort required in modern trials for all drug claims that they considered valid. Such data do not exist for many standard old drugs, as in the case of thirteen anti-parkinsonian drugs called effective by NAS-NRC panels and approved as such by the FDA in the November 7, 1970, *Federal Register.* Indeed, the guidelines for these panels actually instructed them to consider other types of data:

In the deliberations of the Panels, issues will almost certainly arise as to considerations, other than factual evidence, that should be weighed in arriving at judgments on effectiveness. . . . The informed judgment and experience of the members of the Panels is valid evidence contributory to the final decision on the efficacy of a drug.[3]

In some cases, the panels obviously accepted drugs as effective on this basis and this basis alone. Antibiotics experts, for instance, would be entitled to few authoritative statements if they were to limit themselves to the data generated by modern controlled trials. Such trials have not been traditional in infectious disease research, but experts agree nevertheless about the efficacy of certain antibiotics. If such expert judgments have been rendered, and are not contradicted by agency opinion, new trials are apparently not required by the FDA. Hence, decisions are made on the basis of whether the FDA and its advisors feel the need for data from well-controlled trials, not whether such data exist. *Such flexibility is highly desirable,* but the May 8 regulation is self-contradictory nevertheless.

There are other examples of the double standard in FDA or academic judgments on acceptable evidence. Trials whose results favor the new drug over placebo or standard drug tend to be scrutinized in great detail, whereas a negative trial (when a drug appears equal to, or worse than, placebo) is less likely to receive such critical examination. For example, one can, with considerable frequency, detect differences between treatment groups in terms of baseline variables. If enough variables are measured, a few are bound to differ by chance alone. If a trial has been properly designed and strict randomization has occurred, such discrepancies are not ipso facto grounds for rejecting the conclusions of the trial, although discrepancies in regard to a variable known unequivocally to affect response or survival are obviously worrisome. But how often are negative trials scrutinized for such damaging differences?

There are many ways for a trial to come to erroneous conclusions: these include use of the wrong clinical population, too small a sample, measuring the wrong variable, imprecise observations, use of the wrong dose of drug, failure to explore the dose-response relationship, and failure of patients to take the medicine. Furthermore, a negative trial can only conclude that no difference was demonstrated, not that there is no difference. The null hypothesis cannot be proved. Yet it is common to consider a negative trial as important evidence against the drug—perhaps more important than positive evidence. In fact, it should be just the other way around. Several well done positive trials by responsible investigators should be taken as evidence of efficacy, even in the face of a few negative trials, although a large number of the latter would obviously make one wonder about the general utility of the drug or the way in which it was being studied.

Then there is the evaluation of evidence of drug toxicity. For claiming efficacy, controlled trials are quite rightly considered an important anchor to reality, because of the difficulty of predicting the course of the specified patient's disease or symptoms. Patients improve for reasons other than drug effects—because they want to get better (the suggestibility component of the placebo) or because of the healing power of time.

But patients also experience side effects for reasons other than drugs, again for psychological reasons or because of the fortuitous occurrence of dysfunction. It is common, for instance, to find a variety of complaints and laboratory abnormalities during placebo treatment or during no treatment at all.[4] In obtaining well-founded information about drug toxicity, it would be desirable to have placebo control periods, as in trials of efficacy, to facilitate interpretation of the abnormalities observed during active drug treatment. However, much reporting of drug toxicity is in the nature of anecdotal or uncontrolled observations, without placebo data for a standard. Such reporting must not be underestimated; it has been and remains an extremely important means of detecting untoward effects. It must not, on the other hand, be overestimated. *Post hoc ergo propter hoc* data must be taken for what they are worth: circumstantial evidence to be confirmed or rejected by other observations or by epidemiologic or laboratory research. They are rarely proof in or by themselves. One may perhaps justify greater willingness to accept the possibility of harm from a drug than good, but it is at least desirable to be clear about what we are doing and why.

Let us now consider the traditional ways of acquiring evidence in man on the safety and efficacy of drugs.

Anecdotal or "Uncontrolled" Observations

Usually these adjectives are used in a pejorative sense, despite the fact that such observations constitute the oldest method for studying drug actions and remain a mainstay even today. The point too readily forgotten is that they are not, in fact, uncontrolled. The control consists of what the observer believes would have occurred in the absence of the drug. This is the essence of early testing of most drugs, as well as of a great deal of laboratory experimentation of all kinds. The utility of such observations depends upon two things: (1) How valid is the estimate of the baseline or historical control? (2) How easy is it to convince the scientific and regulatory communities of the validity of such controls?

Our older remedies (for example, digitalis, aspirin, anti-epileptic drugs, anti-parkinsonian drugs, most antibiotics, antacids, most dermatological, ophthalmological, and otolaryngological medicaments) have in general been approved on the basis of clinical evidence that was not of the controlled-trial variety. In modern times, L-dopa provides an extremely important example of a drug introduced on the basis of evidence obtained primarily by this type of observation.

The method also remains, thus far, the technique par excellence for uncovering unexpected toxic effects. The letters to the editor in such journals as *Lancet* and the *British Medical Journal* and case reports in journals all over the world testify to the alerting characteristics of observations of this type.

For convincing the scientific community, this method is not as satisfactory as more formal controlled trials and, like all other methods, is subject to false conclusions about both efficacy and toxicity. Chaulmoogra oil was for many years thought to be reasonably effective in the treatment of leprosy, until controlled trials showed it to be little other than a placebo. The evaluation of drugs for therapeutic benefit is risky because many human ailments are not predictable in their course. Even acute leukemia and disseminated malignancy can regress in the absence of any therapy of a recognized sort, so that the proponent of a drug often has difficulty in convincing others that his conclusions from "uncontrolled" trials are warranted.

Still another difficulty is the nonunique character of almost all pharmacologically induced side effects. Even the grotesque seal babies that resulted from the administration of thalidomide were known to occur before and have been described since. Only occasionally (such as in the case of intestinal obstruction or strangulation due to an intrauterine device that has perforated the uterus, or intestinal ulceration from an ondwelling tablet of potassium chloride) is there unequivocal evidence of a cause-and-effect relationship between therapeutic maneuver and untoward events.

As already stated, side effects are more readily attributed to drugs than are beneficial effects. The argument in favor of this practice is that one should bend over backwards to warn physicians and patients of even the remote possibility that a drug might cause harm. Against this point of view is the risk of dissuading physician or patient from the use of a truly superior medication if the drug is undeservedly tarred with the brush of toxicity, particularly if toxicity is also seen after the use of alternative drugs. The listing of unproved side effects also has implications for malpractice suits. One wonders whether at the very least there should not be a caveat as to the degree of confidence with which one may assume that a cause-and-effect relationship exists between a given drug and an alleged side effect.

A major disadvantage of the uncontrolled trial is that it is not good for comparative statements; on the other hand, it is far from useless. The efficacy of penicillin in dramatically altering the course of such diseases as bacterial endocarditis, lobar pneumonia, or syphilis, and the superiority of oral contraceptives to other types of birth control techniques were satisfactorily shown by this type of approach. The oral contraceptives also remind us that controlled trials suitable for comparative purposes may be impossible to do. It is difficult to conceive of a truly randomized allocation of patients to all of the contraceptive techniques now available; even if one could find a subsample of the population that would agree to this kind of trial, they might be so atypical that data obtained on them could not be applied to the population at large. This does not excuse the absence of data on a comparison of one oral contraceptive against another. Such trials could be done without too much difficulty and would have allowed some basis for deciding whether statements about the putative advantages of newer preparations are in fact justified.

Compilation of Anecdotes

This approach also has deficiencies, as exemplified by the National Halothane Study,[5] in which hospital experiences with different anesthetics were analyzed to determine whether halothane gave rise to hepatotoxicity. The major difficulty with a survey of this sort is that a causal relationship between the drugs under study and the recorded morbidity and mortality can never be clearly established because of the confounding of treatment variables with patient and other variables. For instance, if a given anesthetic is routinely used with sicker patients, differences in morbidity and mortality, or even an absence of differences, may be completely meaningless. The argument that different hospitals differ in their philosophy about which agents should be used in such situations scarcely removes this objection.

Another type of compilation of anecdotes includes the national and international registers of spontaneous reports of adverse drug reactions, which in some countries can be compared to consumption figures for the same drugs. It is an interesting commentary on our unbalanced standards of proof that data such as these, for which causality is unproven, tend to be acceptable as evidence of a drug's toxicity or harm, while similar data relating to efficacy or benefit would, if they existed, be totally unacceptable to many.

Challenge-Dechallenge

This is a special type of trial which is neither anecdotal nor a formal controlled comparison of the usual type. It consists of taking someone who has responded with an apparent toxic effect after a medicament and seeing whether readministration of the drug will cause a recrudescence of the difficulty. The results can be quite convincing and often suffice to show that at least some people can respond in this way to the drug. One major drawback is that it is of no use at all in a quantitative sense, that is, in helping one to decide how many people are at risk of the kind of difficulty observed. Another disadvantage is that in ethical, legal, practical, and diagnostic terms its scope is quite limited.

Dose-Response Relationships

The usual way to study dose-response relationships is in a controlled trial, but one can also generate such relationships in relatively untrolled settings. If, for example, oral contraceptives are found in clinical experience to be toxic in proportion to their estrogen content, that fact will bolster those who believe that the pills, as a group, can cause trouble and will suggest that the difficulty may lie with the estrogen component.

Case-Control

The case-control approach is considered by many to be legitimate for toxicological surveys, especially for rare side effects such as the thromboembolic complications of the oral contraceptives. It is generally not considered so legitimate for delineating efficacy.

Retrospective or trohoc studies. In this approach, a control group is chosen to match as closely as possible the target group of patients who have experienced the event in question; the relative frequency with which each group has in the past received the suspected treatment is then determined.

Sometimes valid retrospective matching is almost impossible to achieve. Several studies now going on in Britain show that if one attempts to match women who are taking oral contraceptives with women who are using other types of birth control techniques, there are significant differences in such important variables as socioeconomic class, age, and previous—particularly thromboembolic—disease. For any kind of analysis, even with retrospective stratification, such differences in baseline variables between the groups may render the interpretation of the data extremely difficult.

The possible use of silent genetic markers for substantiating the validity of such case-control observations is intriguing. For example, it was found that women who developed thromboembolism on oral contraceptives had a different distribution in regard to ABO blood types than the population at large. At first sight this suggests some sort of genetic contribution to drug-induced disease. On further analysis, however, it appears that the distribution of blood groups in women who developed thromboembolism on oral contraceptives is not statistically significantly different from what one would expect in the total group of individuals suffering from thromboembolic disease. Since the blood type distribution for the latter is known to be different from that for the total population, such a distribution, rather than the distribution of blood groups in the population at large, represents the appropriate control.

Prospective study with retrospectively identified control group. This is a seldom-used design which has considerable potential. Some years ago it was suggested that an appetite suppressant caused fetal abnormalities. On studying the records of obstetricians who had prescribed the medication and analyzing their data for infants born of such women and infants born of other women in the same practices who had not been treated with the medicament, the two groups were found to have similar frequencies and types of congenital anomalies.[6]

The Comparative Randomized Trial

This approach is relatively new. The biblical trial on diet described in the first chapter of Daniel or the famous trial by James Lind on H.M.S. *Salisbury* on citrus fruits and scurvy[7] are really not trials in the strict modern sense. For example, Lind's experiment would be criticized today because of a difference in baseline variables in his therapeutic groups. He took two patients very sick with scurvy and purposely assigned them to the citrus fruit diet, which he suspected would be beneficial. The therapeutic results were dramatic, but a skeptic could have accused him of using a population destined to improve because they had nowhere to go but up. They might have died, of course, but such trivial points have been known to be completely ignored by a superskeptic with blood in his eye.

Just as the controlled trial is better than the uncontrolled trial for comparative statements, so also the randomized trial can help to equalize the challenge presented to the several treatment groups, in the sense of achieving comparable groups, assembled without bias. Randomization also provides a basis for applying Fisherian statistics and a valid basis for the computation of error. Like every other method, it is not perfect. As one of the modern fathers of the controlled trial, Sir Austin Bradford Hill, has said: "Given the right attitude of mind there is more than one way in which we can study therapeutic efficacy. Any belief that the controlled trial is the only way would mean, not that the pendulum had swung too far, but that it had come right off its hook."

We have discussed several ways in which controlled trials could lead to wrong conclusions. The randomized trial, in its turn, has been criticized recently as suffering from inadequate attention to stratification of patients. If subjects are known to vary on the basis of identifiable baseline characteristics in their response to treatment or in their overall prognosis, it would seem sensible to randomize in a stratified way on these variables. It can be argued that it is only when there is a fairly high correlation between such a predictor and the response to it that matching of any sort is highly useful; [8] moreover, one often does not know which variables are important. Nevertheless, to the extent that important correlations are known to exist, it seems reasonable to believe that the validity and efficiency of clinical trials would be augmented by attention to these details. Certainly, lack of such attention has had serious effects on the interpretation of the results in at least one major recent trial, namely, the University Group Diabetes Program.[9]

In assessing all the evidence about a drug, the question arises of how much pooling of data is allowable. Do protocols used by different investigators have to be exactly the same in order for the data to be pooled for analysis? Is it legitimate to pool the statistical probability values of the different experiments? Are twenty slightly different protocols comparing the same treatments less poolable than the same protocol applied somewhat differently by each center in a multicenter study? If pooling is to be done, should it be applied to the raw data or to the individual analyses?

Inductive Argument from Known Human Models

At times the suspicion that a drug causes serious toxicity in a rare patient can be strengthened by the observation that the drug commonly causes the same effects to a lesser degree. For example, the notion that an occasional person might bleed seriously on acetylsalicylic acid was strengthened by the observation that concealed blood loss of minor degree is routinely seen in most people given modest doses of salicylates. The same sort of analogy can be invoked between the production of mild, asymptomatic hypokalemia, hyperglycemia, or hyperuricemia in many subjects given thiazide diuretics and the occurrence of more significant biological events such as symptomatic hypokalemia, diabetes, or gout in a few patients. Another example is the occurrence of statistically significant, yet usually small, rises in blood pressure in women taking oral contraceptives, predicting—or possibly reflecting—the possibility that an occasional woman will experience a serious rise of blood pressure while taking these agents.

Vital Statistics

Changes in the incidence of certain diseases may give rise to a suspicion that drug-induced trouble is occurring. The German epidemic of phocomelic babies coincident with the introduction of thalidomide is one example of this. The technique is now being utilized to see whether oral contraceptives may be giving rise to an increase in cancer of the breast. Such an approach is usually used for studying toxic effects, but it should also be used for supporting the favorable impact of drugs. It has been suggested, for example, that the recent decline in mortality from hypertension in certain tabulations of vital statistics supports the idea that effective antihypertensive drugs are lifesaving,[10] but other interpretations are possible.[11]

At times vital statistics can provide dramatic evidence of cause-and-effect relationships. The year 1966 showed a dramatic drop in births in Japan. This was a Year of the Dragon, which occurs every twelve years and is, according to oriental astrology, associated with the birth of females who are destined to be bad wives. Apparently a lot of Japanese believe in the association.

Professional Judgment and the Marketplace

Popularity among the public or among physicians is not tantamount to worth, although Peltzman finds that sales of ineffective drugs and new drugs as effective as or less so than other drugs "declined an average of 12.9 percent per year from the first to the fourth year after introduction."[12] Furthermore, there are interesting examples of drugs that have sold well despite an absence of advertising, which suggest that the physician or the patient is not completely lacking in discrimination. It is generally assumed that expert anecdotal judgments are better than non-expert anecdotal judgments, despite the compelling evidence of instances where the practicing doctor has discovered truths that the experts failed to recognize.

CHAPTER IV

WEIGHING THE EVIDENCE

The Concept of Totality of Evidence

In certain instances, one can make a very strong case for linking a drug with certain effects, not because one line of evidence is per se convincing, but because there are many lines of evidence. For example, the oral contraceptives were suspected of causing thromboembolism for the following reasons: case reports of cardiovascular catastrophe in young women, unusual pathological findings in some of these autopsy cases, challenge-rechallenge experiments, the occurrence of cardiovascular toxicity in other therapeutic trials where estrogen alone was administered, the production of clotting factor abnormalities in women given oral contraceptives, the demonstration of decreased venous flow in subjects given hormonal agents, and finally the data from case-control studies.

How Much Imperfection Is Tolerable in a Drug Study?

The perfect trial has never been achieved. Most trials suffer from methodological defects of one sort or another, such as the need to administer other agents than the assigned treatment because of ethically required fail-safe clauses, the breach of the double-blind anonymity by production of side effects by the active agent, differences in baseline variables in treatment groups in the study, and the occurrence of dropouts. The purist would argue that identification of the active agent through the occurrence of toxic effects would automatically invalidate the trial, even if such disclosure did not occur invariably and even if there were not a tidy correlation between side effects and therapeutic impact. The purist would also argue that more than a few dropouts would invalidate a trial. The more practical-minded individual settles for a good deal less than this unattainable ideal. The fact that a study has controls designed into it is usually more important than whether or not all parties are totally blind to the identity of the treatment groups. There is surely a good deal of difference between a trial where dropouts have been modest in number and evenly distributed between the various treatment groups and one where there are either large numbers of dropouts or where there are twice as many dropouts from one treatment group as from another.

Who Shall Evaluate the Evidence?

Any system for weighing evidence will ultimately stand or fall on the honesty and wisdom of the individuals making the judgments. The expert is inclined to believe that people of his own professional background are more likely to make responsible and defensible judgments than are non-experts. The non-experts may, on the other hand, be suspicious of the expert as biased or parochial. Moreover, the idea that experts agree is usually a myth. There are many situations in which one can get respected experts to disagree quite vigorously, as testified by the textbook *Controversy in Internal Medicine*,[1] or by surveys concerning the use of anticoagulants in patients suffering from myocardial infarction or cerebrovascular accidents.

One conclusion that can be drawn from this state of affairs is that one cannot live with experts and one cannot live without them. A more valuable conclusion is that if a respectable minority of professional opinion believes in the utility of a drug, then it ought at least to be available for use by those who believe in it. In fact, the legislative history of the 1962 amendments suggests that this is just what Congress had in mind. For years there was no evidence that drugs for lowering blood pressure prevented morbidity and mortality from cardiovascular events. There is now a body of controlled trial data supporting this point of view. Those who believe that such an effect exists could point out that if mankind had been deprived of the use of such agents until definitive proof came along, thousands of patients would have suffered.

A similar state of affairs may exist with regard to the use of drugs to lower serum cholesterol and triglycerides. No one knows for sure whether such manipulation of blood levels of lipids will prevent new vascular events. There is some rationale for believing that this may be the case, although, as of 1975, controlled trials have so far failed to show unequivocal benefit. Should such medicaments be kept from general use until further expensive and lengthy trials are completed, or should patients and doctors be free to take their chances until the definitive data finally come in?

How Much Is Enough?

Early in the days of the use of reserpine in psychotic patients, a trial was published in which minuscule differences between reserpine and a placebo were shown to be statistically significant because of the large numbers of patients involved in the controlled trial in question. There is a difference between statistical and biological significance. Even a 1 percent difference between a placebo and an active drug can be demonstrated statistically if one is willing to study enough patients.

Three or four well executed trials by people who are expert in a field, with conclusions that are similar, should be enough to demonstrate that a drug is effective. The current FDA position is that two are enough. The accumulation of similar results on thousands of patients often serves merely to provide psychological comfort. If additional trials do in fact provide significant amounts of additional information, they might be useful. If they usually do not, however, it might be worth considering whether the public would not be better off with a combination of earlier marketing and improved post-marketing monitoring, designed to see whether the conclusions generated by early trials by expert physicians can be extrapolated to the population at large, treated by average doctors. Certainly, rare side effects are unlikely to be detected with anything short of huge trials.

The experience with L-dopa is an interesting example of an approach that might well make good sense for other drugs. L-dopa has been a significant advance in the management of Parkinson's disease. Neurologists who worked with the drug were convinced that, regardless of its known hazards or the possibility of unforeseen future difficulties, the compound was too important not to have it generally available. As a result, two NDAs were approved relatively swiftly. In this case, the drug was marketed before the completion of chronic toxicity tests in animals with the understanding that experience with it would be carefully assessed, so that if unforeseen major problems arose the decision could (as with any approved drug) be rapidly reversed. Thus far the decision seems to have been a wise one; by 1975, no unexpected problems had occurred in groups of treated patients monitored for up to five years.

The combination of a moderate amount of impressive clinical experience, coupled with early approval and effective postmarketing monitoring, could be a pattern for the future. It requires, however, postmarketing monitoring of higher quality than has prevailed in the past. For years physicians have voluntarily filed anecdotal reports of untoward effects with journals, detail men, industrial medical departments, the FDA, or the AMA registry of adverse reactions. These data have been of some use, but they do not represent the careful delineation of efficacy and toxicity that could be achieved with a painstaking epidemiologic assessment of the effects of a new drug. Research is urgently needed to develop techniques that would accomplish the desired goals. In addition to monitoring, an educational framework is needed through which the data collected could alert physicians to any nuances in diagnosis, therapy, and toxicity derived from these studies.

Relative Efficacy

From time to time the suggestion is made that the approval of new drugs should take into account the matter of relative efficacy. Indeed, it might be said that when a new drug is introduced, it will be best used if the physician knows where it stands in the hierarchy of drugs available to treat a symptom or disease. In this sense, comparative performance in terms of both efficacy and toxicity is highly important for a judicious choice among medicaments available. The FDA has had a perverse and paradoxical philosophy here; it wants comparative data for approval, dislikes "me-too" drugs, but has usually prohibited comparative claims favorable to the drug from being advertised, even when they are justified.

On the other hand, it is easy to be misled into the stand that a drug must be better than already available drugs in order for it to be marketed or that it is easy to judge what is better. Is erythromycin estolate better than penicillin? Certainly it produces more hepatotoxicity and for many diseases penicillin would be preferred as the antibiotic of first choice, but for certain infections in patients allergic to penicillin it is indeed superior. Is a new drug that cures 20 percent of patients better or worse than a compound that helps 90 percent of the same population but cures nobody? On what yardstick does one compare such different side effects as osteoporosis and agranulocytosis, or increased susceptibility to infection versus peptic ulcer? Can we do without drugs that are no better on the average than those already available, but which—like some drugs in antiepileptic therapy—may be useful for a person who happens not to respond well to the standard drug or who has a toxic reaction from the standard one?

The Appropriate Endpoints

A growing problem surrounds drugs that produce easily measurable effects on endpoints that are not those in which the patient and the clinician are really interested, but whose impact on the condition of real concern is assessable only with great difficulty. For instance, various drugs are known to lower blood cholesterol levels, but no one can be certain that these compounds do in fact prevent degenerative vascular disease, which is the real object of therapy in patients with high blood cholesterol levels. Experience in the field of cancer suggests that compounds that temporarily shrink the size or number of tumors do not necessarily increase life span. In the field of hypertension, on the other hand, at least some drugs that lower blood pressure have indeed been shown to cause a diminution in vascular episodes and a prolongation of life. The recent cooperative study on hypoglycemic drugs has brought into question the safety of oral agents for lowering blood sugar. This study has been both praised and criticized. While the final answer as to the utility of such compounds is not yet known, the results have at the very least raised the specter of inappropriate endpoints misleading manufacturer, patients, and physicians.

Such endpoints have usually been chosen because they are easier to measure than the ones of prime concern. If the results of current studies of oral hypoglycemic agents or cholesterol-lowering drugs should ultimately discredit these compounds, we may see an overall decision to refuse approval to any compound that has not been shown to achieve the prime goal of therapy. To prove that a drug prevents heart attacks is a formidable task. Cooperative studies are required, involving many clinics and many millions of dollars. Such studies are unlikely to be funded by individual companies. Perhaps government underwriting would be appropriate in some cases of this type. Because of the expense of such studies, society will not pay for many of them, and there is always considerable hazard in making decisions on the basis of a single study, no matter how well designed and conducted. We may see the drying up of research in areas such as cholesterol-lowering drugs because of such difficulties and the subsequent absence of informational feedback to the scientists involved in synthesizing and studying such drugs in the laboratory. It could be argued that refusing approval to a drug until theory has been verified by practice is desirable. Yet, as we have already seen, if society had been forced to await the outcome of large-scale trials documenting the benefit of antihypertensive drugs, many thousands of patients, denied these agents, would have died awaiting their approval.

Risk-Benefit Compromises

An important question is how much danger is too much? At one time tranylcypromine was taken off the market, to be reintroduced when psychiatrists came to its defense. This compound, which according to its package insert should be given almost as a last resort in seriously depressed patients, has shown a slow but steady rise in sales in recent years despite the fact that it has not been advertised at all by its manufacturer. Such an occurrence suggests that the drug is used and useful, despite warnings about it. Another example is iproniazid, which was taken off the market because of its alleged capacity to produce hepatotoxicity. Hepatitis is a potentially fatal disease, but so is serious melancholia. There are many who feel that iproniazid was and is the most effective MAO inhibitor available for the treatment of melancholia and that its toxic risks were worth taking in view of its greater therapeutic effect.

Problems of Extrapolation

A separate aspect of how much evidence is enough concerns the question of how much generalization is possible from country to country. There seems little value in repeating preclinical- or clinical-data collection simply for the sake of repeating it, yet one knows that differences do exist between countries in genetics, climate, nutrition, coexistence of other diseases, and so forth. The differential occurrence of jaundice with oral contraceptives in Chile, Finland, and Sweden, as opposed to the rest of the world, suggests real differences from country to country in regard to the clinical performance of these powerful chemicals. If a drug has been shown unequivocally to work in one country, the fact that the drug has potential efficacy should be acceptable to all countries. The problem then becomes one of deciding how much in the way of local evidence is required before one can be confident about the efficacy and safety of the drug in the local population.

Another problem of extrapolation arises with generic drugs. If one manufacturer has shown that a compound works—be it an ethical drug or an over-the-counter preparation—should other manufacturers be required to collect their own clinical trial data to allow them to market the compound or to make the same claims?

Conflicts and Relevance

There are two important areas of conflict generated by society's demand for evidence prior to marketing. The first is between scientific method and ethics. Controlled trials involving placebos, for example, pose ethical problems. It is difficult to defend, from the standpoint of the patient, the use of placebos in an analgesic trial, but easy to defend from the scientific standpoint of evaluating the data, since without placebos finding no difference between the new drug and the old standard one may simply mean that one is dealing with a group of people incapable of discriminating between a good drug and a bad one.

When a patient suffers from a serious disease, there is an ethical problem in trying a new drug when old ones exist which, while imperfect, do a reasonably good job. Utilizing a new drug only in patients in whom standard therapy has failed is not really an answer. Success in such patients is impressive and can justify a trial of a new drug in more responsive individuals, but failure to show a response does not mean that the new drug is ineffective.

It is generally conceded that modern concern with informed consent is a great step forward in terms of the ethics of human experimentation. On the other hand, ethical progress is not necessarily helpful to scientific progress. The obtaining of consent usually results in some loss from lack of volunteers; if the losses are substantial, one is left with the nagging possibility that the sample available for study may not be useful for generalizations at the end of the experiment. There are also some experiments, such as the deliberate use of placebos to obtain therapeutic benefit, that cannot be done at all if fully informed consent is to be obtained.

The second conflict is between the technology of drug assessment and the practice of medicine. It is quite possible that the new developments concerning *substantial evidence* are carrying us further and further away from the real-life situations in which drugs are ultimately to be applied. Certainly most drugs are not given under the circumstances of double-blind technique, obtaining informed consent, hospitalization, the avoidance of other simultaneous therapies, the administration of drugs by experts, and so forth. There are good reasons why the studies upon which the decision to approve marketing is made should be done as they are now, but we should at least recognize that the ultimate use of drugs will be under quite different circumstances and that monitoring of postmarketing performance may become more and more important in assessing the true performance of a drug in practice. Demonstrating drug efficacy is not the same as treating a patient with a disease, and the two should not be confused. As the technology of drug assessment rises in standard and complexity, we must ensure that it fulfills the purpose for which it was developed and does not become an irrelevant charade.

CHAPTER V

ECONOMICS AND
DRUG DEVELOPMENT

An analysis of the rate of introduction of new pharmaceutical products in the United States reveals a substantial decrease over the last fifteen years. For duplicate single products and combination products, the data show that a declining rate was in evidence by the late 1950s, antedating the 1962 amendments to the Food, Drug and Cosmetic Act. For new chemical entities, the fall has occurred primarily since 1962.

Why these changes? Two possible answers to this question are not mutually exclusive. One is that the fantastic earlier output of the pharmaceutical industry preempted many contributions by attacking successfully the easier development problems, and that "post-golden age" research is necessarily less productive because the nuts left to crack are tougher ones.

A second explanation is that the new regulations and new FDA philosophy have generated such expense and such delays in evaluating and approving drugs that the number of successful candidates introduced per year has necessarily shrunk. Mere delays would eventually result in yearly approval rates similar to the old rates; there is no evidence that this catch-up is occurring. As far back as September 12, 1963, at a hearing held before the Subcommittee on Public Health and Welfare of the Committee on Interstate and Foreign Commerce, Congressman Paul Rogers pointed out that there were a good many NDAs that had been filed anywhere from one to five or six years previously. Peltzman has analyzed in economic terms the effects of the 1962 amendments, concluding that they may have been counterproductive.[1]

Bloom has analyzed the available data and concluded that while there has been almost total stifling of new drug approval in a field like the cardiovascular-pulmonary one, the decline has been less remarkable in some other areas, for example, in antibiotics and in the tranquilizer-psychostimulant category. In the area of cancer chemotherapy, there has actually been no decline.[2] Why? Are our techniques for screening drugs or evaluating them better in these fields? Are FDA requirements more lax or flexible in an area like cancer chemotherapy? Can the personal bias of FDA monitors possibly affect the course of events so dramatically?

Clymer has surveyed the economic impact of the new climate of drug development and regulation. He states that in 1968 it actually cost $1,342,000 to bring a new biological to market and somewhat more for a single chemical agent. A year later, Clymer estimated that it took five to seven years and $2.5 to $4.0 million to market one product. For each such product, he estimates that six to ten additional products would "abort along the development path." Making certain assumptions, he calculates that it cost $10.5 million for each successful product, exclusive of the research originally necessary to generate the new compound.[3]

Mund, in a separate analysis, has looked at the research and development costs of the drug industry and concludes that whereas it used to take $1.5 million or so to produce a new single entity, it now takes $15 million.[4]

Mansfield, examining the actual cost and time required in the 1950s and early 1960s for one major drug firm to develop a new chemical entity, found that the average cost was $534,000 during that period, and the total average development time twenty-five months. With a figure of 37 percent successes, the cost of development came to somewhat over $1 million. He notes that an acceptance of Clymer's data would indicate a sixfold increase in the cost of a successful project over nearly a decade, a threefold increase in the length of time required for the project, and a halving of the probability of a given project being successful, with a tenfold increase in total costs per successful new entity. Mansfield further points out that only one-half of this increase would have been foreseen by extrapolating the trends of the fifties and early sixties.[5]

One FDA officer has suggested guidelines for evaluating a new hypolipidemic agent. It has been estimated that an investigation based on these guidelines would cost $2.5 million. Such an estimate does not include the many additional millions required to prove that successful manipulation of blood lipids would indeed favorably affect the course of vascular disease. One wonders to what extent further research in such an area will be pursued in the face of such enormous costs.

In the field of population control, Djerassi calculated in 1970 that a male antifertility agent would require twelve to twenty years and over $6 million to develop, while a luteolytic or abortifacient would take seventeen to eighteen years and over $18 million. He is understandably lugubrious about the incentive for industry to develop new methods of birth control,[6] and his pessimism is borne out by current trends.

It is now clear that the cost of developing a new chemical entity to the stage of NDA approval has been at least doubled since the 1962 amendments (and the regulations adopted thereunder) and that the amendments are responsible for at least a substantial fraction of this increase. There has been a consequent decline in the rate of pharmaceutical innovation achieved with the resources available for pharmaceutical research. It can be concluded that the path to achieving what was intended by Congress should be reexamined to determine whether or not a less costly approach would result in greater benefits to the American public.

PART TWO
Lessons from Other Countries

CHAPTER VI

APPROACHES TO INTERNATIONAL COMPARISONS

So far we have discussed the effects of legislative, scientific, industrial and economic factors on the process of drug discovery and on the technology of drug assessment in the United States. In this section, we shall analyze in detail, using a comparative approach, the ways in which these factors have affected the introduction and use of drugs for the American patient and the practice of medicine in this country.

The United States is not the only country coping with the problems of new drugs; the solutions arrived at in other countries differ in a variety of ways from the American ones. We shall use these facts to examine the performance of American legislation and regulation.

A Survey

It is instructive to examine the difference in speed of introduction of compounds available both in the United States and abroad. Introduction dates in at least one foreign country are available for forty-three of the new single chemical entities marketed in this country during the years 1965–69.

France showed an average lead time of one year; that is, the products were introduced on the average one year sooner than in the United States. Six were introduced in the same year in both countries, three were one year earlier in France, two were two years earlier, two were three years earlier, three were four years earlier, one was seven years earlier, and one was nine years earlier. Six were introduced in France one year after the United States date and three were two years later.

Seven products were introduced in the same year in Germany and the United States, seven were introduced a year later in Germany than in the United States, and ten were introduced one to eight years earlier in Germany. The average lead time was 1.6 years for Germany. England displayed a similar picture, except that the average lead time was even greater—2.1 years.

These products included such drugs as clofibrate, propranolol, cloxacillin and dicloxacillin, allopurinol, azathioprine, deferoxamine, amantadine, dextrothyroxine, carbamazepine, furosemide, ethambutol, methotrimeprazine, amitriptyline, cephaloridine, haloperidol, fentanyl, indomethacin, ethacrynic acid, clomiphene, methacycline, mefenamic acid, doxycycline, doxepin, procarbazine, thiothixene, methaqualone, tolnaftate, hydroxyurea, lincomycin, tybamate, oxazepam, and chlorphentermine.

Such an analysis tells nothing of the degree to which United States regulatory procedures are "protecting" the American public from "poor" drugs introduced abroad but denied access to our market. Nevertheless, it does show a considerable lag in the approval of compounds judged—by their ultimate approval in the United States—to be useful, and to that extent it implies an inferior public performance. As early as 1963, the American Medical Association went so far as to endorse the drug metronidazole (Flagyl) as a uniquely effective trichomonicidal drug to dramatize the fact that the NDA had been languishing for two years at the FDA.

Evidence of this sort provides a circumstantial case for the view that useful new drugs are being unnecessarily delayed or withheld from American patients. However, the whole issue is more complex than this. Ideally it is necessary to examine in detail the individual benefits and losses associated with all the drugs introduced in the United States and foreign countries. The evidence and conclusions to be described in the following chapters are based on a detailed comparison of the United States with the United Kingdom. The latter country was chosen for comparison because it has comparable standards of medical care and a readily accessible pharmacologic and medical literature.

Before embarking on the comparison in detail we must first clarify exactly what is being measured in an international comparison of this type and what the methodology of such a study needs to be.

Methodology

In determining the methodology for examining the effects of legislative and regulatory policies on drug development and usage, one must first find parameters that can be used as measures of effect and then design a study capable of determining the magnitude of such effects if they exist.

Measures of effect. The most obvious effects of regulatory policies are on patterns of drug availability. To measure this, one needs to know the numbers and identities of new drugs and the dates they were introduced.

A specific pattern of drug availability is not of paramount significance in itself; it acquires significance, however, when particular drugs become used in substantial amounts. There are several ways in which one might measure such patterns of drug utilization. Most involve some kind of survey, either through market research organizations, prescription audits, or ad hoc surveys designed to evaluate specific points.

Patterns of drug availability and utilization, while obvious measures, are not the ones of ultimate interest. What we really need to know are the therapeutic outcomes experienced with drugs in the conditions of actual use under different systems of regulation. Unfortunately, few reliable data exist to define therapeutic outcome—either beneficial or hazardous—under conditions of actual drug use; the current state of the art of clinical pharmacology does not yet enable such analyses to be performed rigorously, except in a few instances. This subject will be explored in greater detail in a subsequent chapter.

Legislation and regulation can have other important results. These include effects on the rate of discovery of therapeutically better drugs, on the economics of drug development, and on the practice of medicine. Some of these topics are beyond the scope of the present analysis, while on others there are insufficient data to support a useful analysis. In the present study, we have confined our attention to measures of drug availability, drug utilization, and (where possible) therapeutic outcome.

Study design. There are three possible ways in which to design a study to reveal the effects of legislative and regulatory policies. The first is to study one country vertically in time, comparing the situation before regulatory changes with that afterwards. The converse is a horizontal study, comparing countries possessing different regulatory systems at a given point in time. The third possibility would be to combine these two approaches.

The advantage of following a single country over a period of time is that this excludes the confounding effect of international differences. Unfortunately, a major confounding effect remains—namely, those factors apart from regulatory influences that change with time. These include changes in the process of drug discovery, advances in drug usage and medical science, including changes in non-drug ancillary therapy, and changes in other aspects of medical practice.

Comparing different countries horizontally at a given time has the advantage of removing the time factor with its attendant confounding variables. In this case, the confounding effect of international differences other than regulations is introduced. Industrial practices differ among nations, as do the attitudes and participation of the medical profession (both practicing and academic), the presence or absence of third-party payment schemes for drugs, and levels of medicolegal pressure. All these are inextricably intertwined with regulatory decisions. However, since the process of drug development and discovery is conducted on an international scale and drugs are potentially international commodities, the regulations that control the access of drugs to the market will be among the most important factors in international differences.

The third possibility is to combine the vertical and horizontal approaches, by comparing the temporal effect of a regulatory change in one country with the corresponding effects produced by regulatory changes in other countries. The problem with this is that the nature and the time of introduction of the regulations differ for each country, so that the effect of time as a confounding variable is by no means removed.

Thus, none of the observational approaches is perfect; lacking an experimental approach we are forced to rely on them. In the sections that follow, a horizontal international comparison has been adopted.

It must be kept in mind that the differences to be described are not solely the result of differences in legislative and regulatory policies operating in isolation. In many cases, however, it is possible to discern that differences in regulatory philosophy are a prime cause of differences in drug development and usage.

CHAPTER VII

PATTERNS OF INTRODUCTION OF NEW DRUGS IN BRITAIN AND THE UNITED STATES

There have previously been insufficient data available to make even the most rudimentary international comparisons of the patterns of introduction of new drugs. Industrial and independent sources have pointed to the marketing of certain drugs earlier abroad than in the United States,[1] but these accounts do not include the converse data— drugs that are marketed in the United States earlier than abroad. Furthermore, most of these accounts deal only with those drugs that have so far been marketed in both the United States and a foreign country—that is, drugs that are mutually available—leaving out of consideration those drugs that have been exclusively introduced in the United States or a foreign country. The evidence presented in this chapter deals with both exclusive and mutual marketing and shows that a substantial lag and deficit exist in the introduction of new drugs to the American market.

Americans may be unfamiliar with evidence concerning the efficacy or toxicity of drugs that are unavailable in the United States, or with the use of available drugs for indications that are unapproved here. For that reason a brief review is given of such British-approved drugs or uses which we consider to be of interest for pharmacologic, therapeutic or toxicity reasons.

This chapter consists, therefore, of a comparative tabulation of drugs available for prescription in Britain and the United States, a description of the patterns of introduction of these drugs, and a documented review of the areas where appreciable differences are found

This chapter is an updated and condensed version of W. M. Wardell, "Introduction of New Therapeutic Drugs in the United States and Great Britain: An International Comparison," *Clinical Pharmacology and Therapeutics*, vol. 14 (1973), pp. 773-90. © 1973 by C. V. Mosby Company, St. Louis, Missouri.

to exist between the British and American patterns. This chapter does not deal exhaustively with the complex question of the total therapeutic impact of these differences in terms of benefits and risks to patients in the two countries. It does, however, contain the data on which such a study needs to be based. These wider implications will be explored in the subsequent chapters.

Methods

In this study, the term *new drug* has been defined as a new single chemical entity, excluding vaccines and new salts.

The basic approach was to take a fixed time period and to examine the introduction of new drugs into Britain and the United States during that period. The period chosen was the decade from the beginning of 1962 through the end of 1971, which corresponds to the post-thalidomide decade of drug development. Major developments since 1971 have also been included.

Nine therapeutic areas were selected for study; these were the cardiovascular, diuretic, respiratory, antibacterial, anticancer, central-nervous, anesthetic, analgesic and gastrointestinal areas. Those drugs introduced in these therapeutic areas in either country during the decade defined became the basis of this study. If, however, a drug had been introduced in one of the two countries before 1959, it was excluded from the study, since the object was to deal only with drugs of recent origin. Where a drug had been withdrawn from the market, it was noted with this proviso and discussed, but was excluded from the numerical summary. A similar course was adopted for some drugs encountered during the course of the study which were of medical interest but did not satisfy all the criteria for inclusion. Certain drugs with multiple uses appear in more than one table, but each drug was counted only once in the numerical summary.

There is no official compendium in either country containing the comprehensive data required for this study. Information on the marketing of new drugs in Britain and the United States was obtained in the first place from the appropriate sections of the DeHaen *Non-Proprietary Name Index*.[2] These lists were culled to select only those drugs conforming to the criteria described earlier. Further information, particularly on British marketing dates, was obtained from the publications of Intercontinental Medical Statistics (IMS).[3] With this information as a start, a large amount of data was then obtained from or verified with the manufacturers: fifty pharmaceutical manufacturers, licensees, or marketing companies in the United States, the United Kingdom, and Europe were asked to provide information about the regulatory and international marketing status of drugs owned by them and to clarify international differences in their marketing patterns.

Despite the use of these sources, it is difficult to obtain a completely accurate history of new drug introductions in Britain and the United States, for several reasons. None of the sources is exhaustive: some cover only part of the time period of interest or only part of the market—for example, IMS supplies data on retail but not hospital availability.

Documentation of efficacy (in the form of clinical trial results) for the drugs discussed in this paper was obtained from the American, British, and European medical and scientific literature cited in the notes. Documentation of the frequency and nature of adverse reactions was more difficult. The most frequently occurring adverse reactions are generally documented in the clinical trials literature. However, the small number of patients involved in most clinical trials means that rare side effects will seldom be detected at that stage, and therefore one needs to have access to the results of adverse reaction surveillance systems.

The most comprehensive collection of international adverse reaction data is that compiled by the World Health Organization (WHO) Drug Monitoring Project, details of which are regularly sent to the participating national centers. The only copy of these data existing in the United States is held by the Food and Drug Administration, and a national center can release only that portion of the WHO data that it has originally contributed to the total data bank. Thus, adverse reaction data on drugs not at present available in this country cannot be obtained within the United States by any person outside the Food and Drug Administration.

Recourse was therefore made to secondary sources to document toxicity. Special efforts were made to document those instances in which a noteworthy toxicity problem was known to exist. Sources included the reports of the British Committee on Safety of Drugs, British pharmaceutical manufacturers, articles and correspondence in the British medical literature, and other sources cited in the notes.

Results

The overall statistics will be described before considering individual therapeutic areas and drugs in detail. During the decade 1962–71, 180 new drugs qualified for consideration in these areas (Table 1). For further analysis, one needs to divide these drugs into two classes: *Mutually available drugs* are those which, by the end of 1971, had

Table 1

SUMMARY OF NEW DRUG INTRODUCTIONS IN BRITAIN AND THE UNITED STATES, 1962–1971 [a]

Category	Total Introductions	Mutual						Exclusive				
		U.K. lead		Simultaneous	U.S. lead		Subtotal	U.K.		U.S.		Subtotal
		No. of drugs	Years	(no. of drugs)	No. of drugs	Years		No. of drugs	Years	No. of drugs	Years	
Cardiovascular	17	4	(14)	1	2	(9)	7	10	(42)	0	(0)	10
Diuretic	11	3	(6)	1	1	(1)	5	5	(19)	1	(8)	6
Respiratory	8	0	(0)	0	1	(2)	1	7	(23)	0	(0)	7
Antibacterial etc.	54	16	(44)	3	10	(23)	29	16	(55)	9	(30)	25
Antimitotic etc.	19	4	(9)	1	4	(13)	9	6	(8)	4	(13)	10
CNS	42	10	(26)	4	6	(10)	20	16	(42)	6	(17)	22
Anesthetic	11	3	(10)	1	1	(1)	5	6	(24)	0	(0)	6
Analgesics etc.	9	2	(11)	3	0	(0)	5	3	(6)	1	(0)	4
Gastrointestinal	9	1	(0)	0	0	(0)	1	8	(37)	0	(0)	8
Total	180	43	(120)	14	25	(59)	82	77	(256)	21	(68)	98
Average number of years			2.8			2.4			3.3		3.2	

a In the "years" columns, numbers in parentheses represent drug-years, that is, drug X years, while bottom value is average number of years per drug.

been marketed in both the United States and Britain. For these drugs it is the difference in marketing dates that is relevant, that is, the "lead" or "lag" time, depending on the direction of the difference. *Exclusively available drugs* are those which, by the same date, had been marketed in only one of the two countries. In this case, it is the list of drugs together with marketing dates that is needed.

Eighty-two drugs became mutually available. Of these, fourteen were introduced into both countries during the same year, forty-three were introduced into Britain first with a mean lead time of 2.8 years, and twenty-five were introduced into the United States first with a mean lead time of 2.4 years. Expressed as a single index, among those drugs that have become mutually available, there were 59 "drug-years" of prior availability in the United States, while the corresponding figure for Britain (120 "drug-years") was almostly exactly double.

Ninety-eight drugs became exclusively available. Seventy-seven of these were exclusively available in Britain for an average of 3.3 years each up to the end of 1971, while the corresponding figures for the United States were 21 drugs, for an average of 3.2 years each. In terms of "drug-years" of exclusive availability, the figures were 256 for Britain and 68 for the United States. Thus, expressed either in terms of the number of drugs exclusively available or in terms of "drug-years" of exclusive availability, the British figures are nearly four times those of the United States.

The remainder of this section consists of an examination of five of the nine therapeutic categories in detail and a survey of some others. (The original paper should be consulted for a complete account of all categories.) Drug toxicity has been emphasized; some drugs are discussed solely because of a toxicity or side effect problem.

Cardiovascular drugs (Table 2). Hypolipidemic drugs have not yet received sufficient trial to define the full extent of their benefits and hazards. The position resembles that of hypotensive drugs during the first decade or so of antihypertensive therapy: while evidence of pharmacologic efficacy exists, long-term prophylactic efficacy has not yet been established.[4] We have pointed out earlier that if approval for the prophylactic use of antihypertensive drugs had been withheld until prophylactic efficacy had been scientifically established, such a delay would have represented a major medical disaster. By analogy, on the basis of the evidence currently available, the four-year British lead with clofibrate is a distinct medical advantage, provided that clofibrate is indeed useful in preventing vascular disease. (The recently published results of the U.S. Coronary Drug Project[5] fail to provide support for such usage in patients who have

Table 2

INTRODUCTION OF CARDIOVASCULAR DRUGS

Drug	Date of Introduction U.K.	Date of Introduction U.S.	Lead in Years U.K.	Lead in Years U.S.
Antihypertensive				
Pargyline (Eutonyl, Abbott)	1963	1963	0	0
Methyldopa (Aldomet, M.S.D.)	1962	1963	1	
Bethanidine (Esbatal, B.W.)	1963	—		
Guanoxan (Envacar, Pfizer)	1964	—		
Guanoclor (Vatensol, Pfizer)	1964	—		
The β-blockers[a]	1965	—		
Debrisoquin (Declinax, Roche)	1967	—		
Clonidine (Catapres, Boehringer)	1971	—		
β-adrenoreceptor antagonist				
Propranolol (Inderal, I.C.I.)	1965	1968	3	
Practolol (Eraldin, I.C.I.)	1970	—		
Oxprenolol (Trasicor, Ciba)	1970	—		
Antiarrhythmic				
Bretylium tosylate[b, c] (Darenthin, B.W.)	1959[d]	—		
β-blockers[a] other than propranolol	1970	—		
Anti-anginal, vasodilator and miscellaneous				
Isoxuprine (Vasodilan, Mead Johnson)	1963	1959		4
Prenylamine[c] (Synadrin 60, Hoechst)	1961	—		
Benziodarone[b, e] (Cardivix, Genatosan)	1962	—		
Trimetazidine[b] (Vastarel, Servier)	1964	—		
The β-blockers[a]	1965	—		
Verapamil (Cordilox, Harvey)	1967	—		
Moxisylyte[b] (Opilon, Warner)	1968	—		
Hypolipidemic				
Dextrothyroxine (Choloxin, Flint)	1961	1967	6	
Cholestyramine (Cuemid, M.S.D.)	1970	1965[f]		5
Clofibrate (Atromid-S, I.C.I.)	1963	1967	4	

[a] Listed here but counted under a different heading in the numerical summary.

[b] International Nonproprietary Name.

[c] Listed but does not satisfy all criteria for inclusion in numerical summary.

[d] As antihypertensive.

[e] Subsequently withdrawn. Listed but not included in numerical summary.

[f] Not approved as hypolipidemic in U.S.

already suffered a coronary occlusion.) Cholestyramine, while available in the United States, was not approved for use as a hypolipidemic agent until August 1973.

In economic terms, the following example is highly relevant here. Peltzman [6] calculated the economic effects of introducing a hypothetical drug therapy in 1970 which could gradually reduce the death rate from all heart disease by 10 percent by 1980. He estimated that a delay of only two years in the introduction of such an agent would cost the United States $2.5 billion.

Of the β-blocking drugs, propranolol (Inderal) is still the only one available in the United States. Furthermore, the approved uses of propranolol in the United States were, until 1973, restricted to cardiac arrhythmias of specified types: pheochromocytoma and hypertrophic subaortic stenosis.[7] Abroad it has two major additional indications: angina and hypertension. These two additional indications have been well documented in both the British and American literature.[8] The advantages and side effects of the β-blockers in these conditions are clearly defined, and American restrictions on the use of propranolol have a definite therapeutic impact. The evidence for the efficacy of propranolol in angina and hypertension is unequivocal, while the unwanted effects are pharmacologically predictable, dose-dependent, and manageable, given the precautions associated with any potent therapy.

As we shall show, the β-blockers have had considerable impact in the management, by British experts, of both angina and hypertension. Furthermore, descriptions advocating the use of propranolol in angina appear in the 1971 *AMA Drug Evaluations*[9] and in at last one major American textbook of medicine, in which the author observed that, "[in] the opinion of some experienced workers, the introduction of propranolol in the treatment of angina represents the most significant advance in medical management since the advent of nitroglycerin." In the same textbook, the use of propranolol in the treatment of hypertension is described in 1971.[10] Despite this, propranolol was not approved for the treatment of angina in the United States until 1973, and as of 1975 was still not approved for the treatment of hypertension. This situation is reminiscent of that with the local anesthetic lidocaine, which was recommended and used for cardiac arrhythmias for some years—and indeed was a drug of first choice [11] —before being approved for this purpose in the United States in 1971.

The medicolegal consequences to an American physician of using an available drug for a nonapproved purpose are discussed later. The consequences to his patients may be even more formidable, since the manufacturer cannot provide instructions for proper use, warnings, dose recommendations, or sometimes even appropriate dosage forms of the drug for such nonapproved purposes. Prior to the approval of lidocaine as an anti-arrhythmic, the available dosage forms were inappropriate and no directions on use for arrhythmias could be supplied, despite the fact that this had become the drug of first choice for patients with post-infarction ventricular arrhythmias (including, it is reported, a former President of the United States).

In the family of β-blockers, a number of subsequent members have appeared. Nearly a dozen newer members had been introduced in other countries by June 1975, while propranolol remained the only one available in the United States. The newer β-blockers are of interest pharmacologically because most of them differ from propranolol in having one or more of the following features which are of potential value to some patients: intrinsic sympathomimetic activity, cardioselectivity, and less membrane-depressant activity. These properties can result in less cardiac-depressant action than is produced by propranolol, as well as less tendency to produce bronchospasm; such drugs will theoretically be safer than propranolol in patients with heart failure or asthma. In the United States propranolol is specifically contraindicated in such patients, who therefore have no alternative therapy available.

Practolol was the first of the newer β-blockers, and the first to possess the desirable property of cardioselectivity. It has been shown to be effective in the treatment of angina,[12] hypertension,[13] and arrhythmias.[14] Oxprenolol, which possesses intrinsic sympathomimetic activity, has also been shown to be effective in the treatment of angina [15] and hypertension,[16] and comparable evidence exists for most of the other new β-blockers. As predicted from the way in which they differ pharmacologically from propanolol, both practolol and oxprenolol have less cardiac [17] and bronchial [18] side effects than propanolol. They can therefore be used in some of these patients with asthma or heart failure who do not tolerate propranolol and for whom in the United States propranolol is specifically contraindicated.[19] Similar evidence of relative benefits over propranolol is accruing for certain other newer β-blockers.

Against these advantages must be offset the risks of using a new agent that has not been as widely used in man as propranolol and whose hazards are less well known. Practolol, the first cardioselective β-blocker, was found to produce peculiar skin, retroperitoneal and eye changes that have been serious in a few patients and have led to cessation of promotion by the manufacturer. Even in the United States, where the drug was being widely studied in patients under the IND procedure, it is being replaced by other cardioselective agents. This drug is thus an important example that illustrates both the complex risk-benefit decisions that arise with new drugs and the need for these decisions to be made by the physician with full knowledge of both the patient's needs and the drug's effects.

The hazards of long-term use of the β-blockers, particularly the newer ones, are not yet known. Large-scale clinical investigation of all β-blockers other than propranolol was once temporarily halted in the United States, pending elucidation of a suspicion that they might produce tumors in one strain of mouse. The scientific basis for this suspicion was not fully accepted outside the United States and wide use of β-blockers continues abroad. This is clearly a situation in which large international differences have developed in the interpretation of animal toxicity tests. It is regrettable that all the evidence in this kind of situation cannot be made openly available to the scientific community, as is customary in other spheres of science. The main argument against the newer β-blockers appears to be one of guilt by association, the association in this case being similarity of chemical structure. Even if it were ultimately shown that the newer β-blockers actually could produce tumors in an animal strain, it should be remembered that this type of attribute is by no means unique, nor is it necessarily more sinister than the alternative possible hazards that accompany the use of any drug. It is one further example of the well-known problem of extrapolating from animal tests to man.[20] Many drugs known to produce tumors or leukemias in animals are already widely used in man—for example, estrogens, isoniazid,[21] metronidazole,[22] and griseofulvin.[23] Even agents capable of producing cancer in man are extensively used when necessary—for example, immunosuppressants and ionizing radiation. In terms of numbers of patients harmed, the toxicity that even these latter agents actually cause in man is small compared with that caused by more familiar agents such as digitalis, gold injections, corticosteroids, certain antibiotics, anticoagulants, and anti-inflammatory analgesics. The important point is that this type of risk-benefit decision should ultimately be made by single physicians for individual patients, rather than by a regulatory agency for society as a whole. There exist identifiable groups of patients who obtain great benefit from certain β-blockers in angina or hypertension, yet who cannot tolerate propranolol. For some of these patients, common sense could clearly indicate use of the newer β-blockers. Even a demonstrably hazardous one could be indicated if it had compensatory advantages. The need to make decisions of this type has long been commonplace in medicine. The only new element in this situation is that the decisions are now being taken by committees on behalf of all physicians and all patients.

A further important issue has been raised by the nature of the chemical structures of the newer β-blockers. In the United States, the regulatory response has been to require further carcinogenicity tests of the newer β-blockers in animals. However, the number of *humans* in other countries currently receiving these drugs is already many times greater than the number of animals that could be realistically contemplated for toxicity tests. Logically, therefore, further animal tests at this stage, although of academic interest, appear to be not only (as we shall see in Part Three) uninterpretable but unnecessary as well: if further information is deemed necessary, money would be better directed towards obtaining or improving the data available from scientific surveillance of patients already receiving these drugs in other countries. At the same time, these drugs should be marketed for valid indications in the United States, provided that long-term surveillance can be instituted. Whether effective outpatient surveillance exists at all in the United States is an important point to be discussed later.

Of the other antihypertensive drugs available exclusively in Britain, we shall first consider the adrenergic-neurone blocking drugs bethanidine (Esbatal) and debrisoquin (Declinax). Bethanidine is a classic example of a drug which is pharmacologically very similar to a slightly longer-established drug (guanethidine) but in which relatively small differences can be useful in practice. Bethanidine differs pharmacokinetically from guanethidine in having a quicker onset and shorter duration of action. It also causes much less diarrhea, and many patients greatly prefer bethanidine over guanethidine. In one excellent crossover trial which compared bethanidine, guanethidine, and methyldopa, bethanidine had, for a comparable degree of blood-pressure control, the lowest incidence of side effects necessitating discontinuation of therapy and was the drug most preferred by the patients.[24] Bethanidine is also useful when rapid reduction of blood pressure is required and is easier to use than guanethidine because of its flexibility of control.[25] Debrisoquin is somewhat similar to bethanidine,[26] but less widely used. There is little to choose between guanethidine, bethanidine and debrisoquin in terms of efficacy and safety, but the availability of several agents makes it easier to tailor a patient's therapy to his individual needs and sensitivities. Since bethanidine and debrisoquin are no more hazardous than guanethidine and in many instances are preferable to it because of fewer side effects, more convenience, and greater flexibility of dose schedules, they are useful additions to the range of adrenergic-neurone blocking drugs, and their unavailability to the American public represents a loss.

Guanoxan (Envacar) and guanoclor (Vatensol) are additional members of the adrenergic-neurone blocking group exclusively available in Britain. Both compounds are very effective antihypertensive agents.[27] However, they have not achieved the wide usage of bethanidine and guanethidine because they have a relatively high incidence of side effects, particularly, in the case of guanoxan, liver toxicity. Nevertheless, because of their effectiveness they have been useful in patients who fail to respond satisfactorily to other agents.[28]

It might be argued that the benefits offered by some of the newer antihypertensive agents available exclusively in Britain are offset by the availability there of more toxic compounds. Such an argument has been advanced by the Food and Drug Administration with respect to guanoxan.[29] To support this argument, it would need to be shown that guanoxan is being used inappropriately in Britain. As just shown, guanoxan is a useful drug to have in reserve when other powerful agents have failed. The high incidence of biochemical abnormalities of liver function in patients on long-term guanoxan therapy became apparent soon after its marketing and is well known, partly as a result of a specific warning letter sent by the company to all physicians and partly by inclusion of this information in the product literature. It is obvious that the optimum use of this agent would restrict it to those few patients who fail to respond to other agents. Direct information on the way in which guanoxan is used in Britain is not available, but circumstantial evidence can be adduced in the form of sales figures supplied by market research organizations and by the pharmaceutical companies. From market research data, the total amount of guanoxan supplied to retail pharmacies in Britain during 1971 was compared with the total amount of methyldopa supplied.[30] For the purpose of this comparison, sales of the various dose forms were converted to the weight of the drug. The weight of methyldopa supplied was more than 4,000 times the weight of guanoxan. Assuming that the average daily dose of guanoxan is one-tenth that of methyldopa, the number of patient-days of guanoxan therapy supplied was less than 0.25 percent of that of methyldopa therapy. Information provided at the author's request by the Pfizer Corporation corroborates this picture: the value of total world sales of guanoxan was stated to be less than 1 percent of the value of the United States market alone for all antihypertensive drugs.

These data, while not proving that guanoxan is promoted and prescribed responsibly in Britain, are consistent with that view. Certainly it is difficult to argue a priori that guanoxan is being over-promoted and used in irresponsibly large amounts in Britain. It is similarly difficult to accept the FDA's contention that the American patient is better off by being deprived of it.

Furthermore, one must also balance against the toxicity of guanoxan the fact that some hypotensive agents available exclusively in the United States, while possessing less toxicity than guanoxan, have subsequently been judged only "possibly effective" in the drug efficacy study performed for the FDA.[31] Guanoxan is a powerful hypotensive drug, the severest side effects of which are visible and reversible. In contrast, the main adverse reaction associated with use of drugs that are not fully effective is failure to control the damaging effects of hypertension, which may be subtle, but are sometimes catastrophic and irreversible. It could be argued that the British patient was in principle better off in at least having access to a powerful agent with frequent, visible side effects than the American patient was in having available instead less effective therapies for a hazardous disease. The wider implications of this type of argument will be explored later.

Clonidine (Catapres) is a relatively new and effective antihypertensive agent, exclusively available in Britain until 1974, and its place in hypotensive regimens is still evolving.[32] Clonidine resembles methyldopa and reserpine in terms of efficacy and in its relative lack of orthostatic side effects. It offers a useful alternative to methyldopa or reserpine because its spectrum of side effects is different.[33] It is also useful in hypertensive emergencies.[34]

In lower dosage and under a different brand name (Dixarit), clonidine is also marketed as a prophylactic agent against migraine. Some clinical trials have shown that the drug is effective for certain patients, its main effect being a modest lowering of the frequency of severe attacks.[35] Further trials are needed to assess fully the value of clonidine in this situation, but for those American patients who could benefit from it, its restriction from the market here already seems to be a poor judgment.

Benziodarone (Cardivix) is of interest because it was the first agent to be withdrawn from the British market for toxicity reasons following the establishment of the register of adverse reactions by the Committee on Safety of Drugs.[36] This compound was introduced as an anti-anginal agent, although the evidence for its efficacy, like that of all anti-anginal compounds except nitrogylcerin and the β-blockers, is weak. By 1964, two-and-one-half years after its introduction, eleven cases of jaundice occurring in patients taking the drug had been reported to the Committee on Safety of Drugs or to the manufacturer.[37] Benziodarone was then voluntarily withdrawn from the market by the manufacturer. (In Britain, all such compliance by the industry was voluntary prior to September 1971, but compliance was virtually total.)

Respiratory drugs (Table 3). All but two of the drugs in this category were still exclusively available in Britain by the end of 1971, but two of these were released in the United States in 1973. The most significant of these, cromolyn sodium (Intal), became available in the United States five-and-one-half years after its approval in Britain, the United States being then the fifty-sixth country in the world in which this drug became available. Cromolyn sodium is the first of a unique new class of agents that prevent the release from mast cells of the chemical mediators of immediate hypersensitivity reactions. It has a modest but definite place in the prophylaxis of allergic asthma. The patients who are likely to respond and the nature and

Table 3
INTRODUCTION OF RESPIRATORY DRUGS

Drug	Date of Introduction		Lead in Years	
	U.K.	U.S.	U.K.	U.S.
Sputum liquifiers				
Acetylcysteine (Mucomyst, Mead Johnson)	1965	1963		2
Bromhexine (Bisolvon, Boehringer)	1968	—		
Bronchodilators				
Isoetharine[a] (Dilabron, also in Bronkometer, Breon)	1970	1961[b]		
Metaproterenol (Alupent, Boehringer)	1962	1973	11[d]	
Proxyphylline[c] (Thean, Astra)	1967	—		
Acefylline[c] piperazine (Etophyllate, Delandale)	1968	—		
Albuterol (Ventolin, A&H)	1969	—		
Terbutaline (Bricanyl, Astra)	1971	—		
Antiallergic				
Cromolyn sodium (Intal, Fisons)	1968	1973	5[d]	
(Rynacrom,[d] Fisons)	1971	—		

[a] Listed but does not satisfy all criteria for inclusion in numerical summary.
[b] Not available as a single drug.
[c] International Nonproprietary Name.
[d] Listed here but not counted in numerical summary.

amount of benefit obtained, which can include reduction of steroid requirements, were well defined in both the foreign and the American literature several years ago.[38] Recently, cromolyn sodium was marketed in a new dosage form for nasal insufflation in the prophylaxis of seasonal allergic rhinitis. Although few published studies exist on this topic, it appears to be effective in reducing nasal obstruction, rhinorrhea, and antihistamine consumption, but less effective in reducing sneezing and itching.[39]

The absence of cromolyn sodium from the American market for five-and-one-half years after its introduction in Britain represents a definite disadvantage to those allergic asthma sufferers who derive clear benefit from this agent.

The β-agonist bronchodilators orciprenaline (metaproterenol—Alupent), salbutamol (albuterol—Ventolin) and terbutaline (Bricanyl) differ in several ways from the prototype of their series, isoproterenol. They are more reliably absorbed when administered by mouth; they have a longer duration of action; and—most important—they are relatively bronchoselective. That is, all three produce less cardiac stimulation for a given bronchodilator effect than does isoproterenol. Salbutamol is the most bronchoselective and metaproterenol the least so of the three.[40] Metaproterenol was the first of these bronchoselective bronchodilators to become available in the United States. It was marketed in 1973, eleven years after its introduction in Britain.

Isoetharine has properties similar to those of the orally active, bronchoselective β-agonists described above.[41] Although at first sight it appears to have been marketed in the United States a decade before its marketing in Britain, the marketing history in this case is complex and atypical. Isoetharine was marketed in the United States in 1961, but not as a separate substance: it was combined with an α-agonist (phenylephrine) and an antihistamine (thenyldiamine) in dose forms for inhalation only (Bronkometer and Bronkosol, Breon). Subsequently, the drug efficacy study of the National Academy of Sciences rated Bronkometer and Bronkosol "effective, but" and then "ineffective as a fixed combination." Isoetharine was not, by 1971, available in the United States without the antihistamine, nor is it available in an oral dose form. In 1971, isoetharine was introduced onto the British market as the single substance (Numotac, Riker).

These bronchoselective sympathomimetic bronchodilators are effective and are, in terms of acute cardiac side effects, safer than isoproterenol. However, it should be realized that the true worth of any bronchodilator in the therapy of asthma has not been fully established; questions of both long-term efficacy and safety are as yet unresolved.[42]

In the early and mid-1960s there was a large increase in mortality from asthma in Britain, especially among young people. This was attributed to the excessive use of sympathomimetic bronchodilator inhalers, obtained either on prescription or over the counter. The exact mechanism for these deaths has not been clearly established, but it appears that several bronchodilator compounds were involved and that the excess mortality could not be attributed solely to orciprenaline, the only one of the three newer agents available at that time. Furthermore, the rise in death rate began before sales of orciprenaline became significant. Conolly, Davies, Dollery and George reviewed the sequence of events involved in this epidemic and the four possible mechanisms that have been postulated to explain it.[43] Stolley presented indirect evidence supporting a fifth possible cause, the availability of higher-strength preparations of isoproterenol in Britain and other countries which experienced the increased mortality.[44] These hypotheses are not mutually exclusive, and all involve excessive use of the bronchodilators. In the present state of knowledge in this area one can say that Britain has available some bronchodilators with very probable therapeutic advantages over isoproterenol, and that new drugs per se were not responsible for the excess asthma mortality of the 1960s. As will be discussed later, this episode is attributable more to the absence at that time of adequate surveillance procedures than to laxity in the introduction of any new drug or dose form.

Antibacterial drugs. Among the antibacterial drugs exclusively available in 1971 in the United Kingdom, the most important was co-trimoxazole (Septra, Bactrim), the one-to-five combination of trimethoprim and sulphamethoxazole. Trimethoprim is an inhibitor of the enzyme dihydrofolate reductase, having particular affinity for that enzyme in bacteria and certain protozoa. Trimethoprim, therefore, blocks the pathway to folate at a point separate from but in sequence with the sulfonamides. The ingredients of co-trimoxazole act synergistically, possess an antibacterial spectrum wider than the sulfonamides, and, furthermore, the combination is bactericidal. The discovery of trimethoprim has been described as "an important landmark in the history of chemotherapy" and its introduction in synergistic combination with the sulfonamides as "a major advance in therapeutics."[45] Its effectiveness and widespread use in treating many infections, including those of the urinary tract, have been documented.[46] Of greater importance, however, are situations where other agents have failed and where co-trimoxazole may prove lifesaving. This was demonstrated early in the history of the compound:

in septicemias due to Proteus [47] and Escherichia [48] and systemic nocardiosis,[49] in all of which other agents had failed. Other infections responsive to co-trimoxazole include typhoid fever, gonorrhea, staphylococcal osteomyelitis, some fungal infections in addition to systemic nocardiosis, and some protozoal infections, including malaria. The United States was the 106th country to approve this compound for the market. It was approved in the United States in August 1973, some five years after its introduction into Britain, with approval limited to the treatment of urinary tract infections.

Despite the obvious importance of this agent and despite the fact that it had been available in Britain since 1968, this compound was much delayed in receiving acknowledgment in the United States. It received no mention in *AMA Drug Evaluations* (1971),[50] the *Cecil-Loeb Textbook of Medicine* (1971),[51] or *Drugs of Choice 1972-1973.*[52] The low awareness of this agent among physicians in one American academic center as long as four years after its introduction in Britain will be described later.

Fusidic acid (Fucidin), marketed in 1962 in Britain but not in the United States, has a steroidal structure resembling cephalosporin P_1, and is active orally as well as parenterally. Its particular utility is in the treatment of staphylococcal infections.[53] It is used alone and in combination with other antibiotics, particularly when the organism is resistant to the penicillinase-resistant penicillins or the patient is hypersensitive to penicillin. Controlled trials with other active agents are conspicuously absent in antibacterial chemotherapy. However, useful results have been demonstrated in miscellaneous staphylococcal infections, including septicemias and pneumonias,[54] and particularly in staphylococcal osteomyelitis,[55] which is the main indication for this drug.

With the alternatives now available, fusidic acid is probably of less importance today than in 1962, when it was first introduced. It remains nevertheless an agent of first choice abroad for some serious staphylococcal infections, in particular staphylococcal osteomyelitis. It is still not available in the United States.

Antitubercular antibiotics. The main advances of the decade were rifampin, ethambutol and ethionamide. Rifampin is undoubtedly the most significant of these and is widely regarded as the most important antitubercular agent since the discovery of isoniazid. Only ethambutol became available simultaneously in both countries; rifampin and ethionamide were released respectively two and three years earlier in Britain.

The medical effects of these delays in the United States would have been felt by those patients who experienced side effects to more toxic existing agents, or by those whose organisms were resistant. There is still appreciable mortality from tuberculosis in the United States—6,292 deaths in 1968.[56] All available therapy for tuberculosis has appreciable hazards, rifampin being one of the least toxic of the highly effective agents. There is little room for complacency in the United States about the delay in the introduction of effective new antitubercular therapies. The United States was the fifty-first country in which rifampin became available.

Of interest as a historical analogy is an analysis of the economic benefits of the introduction of streptomycin, PAS, and isoniazid. Peltzman has estimated that a two-year delay in the introduction of these agents would have cost the United States $2 billion with an excess mortality of 13,000 people.[57]

Centrally acting drugs. In this category there are several groups to be considered.

Psychotropic drugs. Haloperidol is one compound for which delay (six years) in reaching the American market can be considered noteworthy, since it is the first member of a new therapeutic class. This agent is a useful alternative to the phenothiazines but its advantages, while positive, are difficult to quantify. It does, however, appear to have unique activity in controlling the symptoms of the Gilles de la Tourette syndrome[58] and can be considered to be of major importance to the few patients suffering from this condition.

Although lithium salts were only approved a year later in the United States than in Britain for the treatment of manic-depressive illness, the United States was the fiftieth country in which this drug became available.

Anticonvulsants. The anticonvulsants sulthiamine (Ospolot) and carbamazepine (Tegretol) are useful agents for some patients,[59] and this fact alone is sufficient to justify their availability. Sulthiamine is not available in the United States. Carbamazepine was introduced into Britain in 1963. It is effective in the treatment of trigeminal neuralgia and is also useful in epilepsies, particularly psychomotor epilepsy refractory to other agents.[60] It is approved for use in grand mal and temporal lobe epilepsies in Britain. In 1968, carbamazepine was approved for use in trigeminal neuralgia in the United States, but it was not approved for use in epilepsy until 1974.

Other centrally acting drugs. Fenfluramine (Ponderax) is an interesting example of an appetite suppressant which has a slight sedative, rather than stimulant, action.[61] In the treatment of obesity, its only indication, fenfluramine has efficacy comparable to that of the amphetamine-like agents.[62] Although dependence can be demonstrated after chronic administration, the drug has not thus far proved sufficiently attractive to cause significant abuse.[63] A working party of the British Medical Association, reporting in 1968 on amphetamines and amphetamine-like preparations, stated with regard to the treatment of obesity that "of the compounds available, fenfluramine seems to have the least undesirable side effects." [64] Furthermore, fenfluramine has been shown not to antagonize the actions of antihypertensive agents, a unique property and an important consideration in patients who are both obese and hypertensive. At least two studies have shown that fenfluramine actually potentiates the action of antihypertensive drugs.[65] It was introduced into the American market in 1973, nine years after its British marketing date.

In view of all the concern that has been shown about amphetamines, it is difficult to postulate that the United States has gained by excluding for nearly a decade an agent whose addictive potential appears to be minimal and which possesses the other advantages listed.

Nitrazepam (Mogadon) is a benzodiazepine that has come to be widely used as an outpatient hypnotic abroad, having been marketed in Britain in 1965. Its main feature as a hypnotic is its safety in acute overdose; deaths from suicide attempts with this compound are very rare.[66] Its hypnotic properties appear to be similar to those of flurazepam, the first benzodiazepine hypnotic to be introduced on the American market some six years after nitrazepam was introduced in Britain. In addition, nitrazepam is one of the more effective anticonvulsants of the benzodiazepine series and is the most effective agent available for the treatment of myoclonic seizures.[67]

The exceptional safety of nitrazepam in acute overdosage has been long established. Matthew et al. contrasted the clinical result of overdosage with nitrazepam to that seen with other hypnotics in over 1,000 patients seen at a regional poisoning treatment center. They noted that the effect of nitrazepam poisoning was completely different from that seen with other agents: "Of 102 [patients] poisoned by nitrazepam none was deeply unconscious and no patient was unconscious for more than twelve hours. Intensive cardiorespiratory care was not required and no complications occurred in their management. This supports the findings of Matthew and his colleagues in their limited series of 27 patients and there remains no authenticated record of death due to nitrazepam poisoning." [68] The safety of nitrazepam in overdosage has led some British physicians to advocate that it should replace other hypnotics for outpatients.[69] In New Zealand, such action was officially recommended by the National Poisons Centre in a letter to all physicians in that country, pointing out that the exclusive use of nitrazepam or oxazepam as hypnotics in outpatients "might abolish most of the serious problems associated with overdosage of hypnotics." By 1971 nitrazepam was the most frequently prescribed hypnotic in New Zealand, accounting for one-third of all hypnotic use.[70]

The situation in the United States was very different. No benzodiazepine was approved for use as a hypnotic until the marketing of flurazepam in 1971. Thus, if an American physician had wanted to prescribe the then-available benzodiazepines such as diazepam (Valium) or chlordiazepoxide (Librium) as hypnotics, he would have been—and still is—officially discouraged from doing so. Although a physician faces no direct legal sanction in using drugs for such unapproved purposes,[71] it is generally agreed that such action would not favor his cause in a malpractice suit.

The implications of this particular difference between British and American practice are not trivial, although in the absence of direct information one is forced to use circumstantial evidence. During 1968 and 1969, the latest years for which full data are available, 1,514 accidental poisoning fatalities due to sedatives and hypnotics were reported in the United States, of which twenty-one were children under five years of age.[72] This figure is extremely conservative—indeed a gross underestimate—because of under-reporting to the National Clearinghouse. Extrapolated to the five-year period for which a benzodiazepine hypnotic was approved in Britain but not the United States, this figure implies that there were at least 3,700 deaths, including 50 children, from sedatives and hypnotics in the United States during this period. The corresponding figures for barbiturates alone were 1,890 deaths, including 45 children. Most of these deaths would have been preventable if a safe sedative had been involved. Judging from the New Zealand figures for nitrazepam usage, one-third of the deaths due to hypnotics would have been preventable if there had been earlier introduction, vigorous promotion and official endorsement, rather than discouragement, of a benzodiazepine or a comparable, safe hypnotic. The point is obvious. Introduction of a new drug that produced fatalities anywhere approaching this magnitude would be regarded as a major disaster, but the undoubted occurrence of deaths through failure to introduce a drug has so far gone unremarked. It would not take many examples of this type to show that earlier introduction of some new drugs might more than counterbalance all the new drug toxicity of the past decade. It is worth noting here that if all deaths from hypnotics and sedatives were regarded as preventable over the five-year period, the potential reduction in American fatalities would slightly exceed in numbers the total excess asthma mortality previously described for Britain.

The nitrazepam example also illustrates the point made earlier about the difficulty of separating regulatory from industrial causes. The company concerned (Roche) had not applied to market nitrazepam as a hypnotic in the U.S. Both direct industrial decisions and the indirect effects of regulatory policies contributed to this, but elucidating the relative roles of each has defied extensive enquiries by the authors. The high cost of obtaining approval of a new drug application in the U.S. and the lack of acceptability, until very recently, of any but American clinical experience undoubtedly play an important role in industrial decisions. Industrial decisions are themselves influenced by the regulatory atmosphere.

While on the subject of poisoning, the example of deferoxamine (Desferal) is relevant. This chelating agent is the only specific antidote available for the treatment of iron poisoning. It was introduced in Britain in 1962. Three years later, some American authors reporting favorable studies with this compound prefaced their paper in the American literature with the remark: "Currently there is no effective therapy for acute iron poisoning. . . ." [73] It was a *further* three years before deferoxamine became available in the United States.

The reported incidence of deaths from severe iron poisoning, that is, in patients who are in coma or shock, has fallen dramatically in the past two decades.[74] Part of this fall is due to improvement in nonspecific supportive therapy. Deferoxamine has undoubtedly played an important part, although its exact role cannot be quantified because of the concomitant changes in ancillary therapy. The available data, however, provide no grounds for complacency over the six-year delay in the introduction of this useful antidote.

Gastrointestinal drugs (Table 4). Two therapeutic agents have been derived from licorice: carbenoxolone sodium and deglycyrrhizinated licorice. Carbenoxolone (Biogastrone) [75] is the semi-synthetic semi-succinate of β-glycyrrhetinic acid, which is a derivative of glycyrrhizic acid, a glycoside extracted from licorice.[76] There is no doubt that carbenoxolone accelerates the rate and amount of healing of gastric ulcers in a substantial proportion of patients.[77] Results achieved by carbenoxolone in ambulant outpatients are equivalent to those obtained by bed rest in hospital. Carbenoxolone is by no means an ideal treatment. Although it accelerates the healing of ulcers, it

Table 4
INTRODUCTION OF GASTROINTESTINAL DRUGS

Drug	Date of Introduction		Lead in Years	
	U.K.	U.S.	U.K.	U.S.
Peptic ulcer				
Carbenoxolone[a] (Biogastrone, Berk)	1963	—		
Deglycyrrhizinated licorice[b] (Caved-S, Tillots)	1963	—		
Gefarnate[a] (Gefarnil, Crookes)	1968	—		
General				
Metoclopramide (Maxolon, Beecham)	1967	—		
Mebeverine (Colofac, Duphar)	1967	—		
Lactulose (Duphalac, Duphar)	1969	—		
Diagnostic				
Pentagastrin (Peptavlon, ICI)	1967	—		
Secretin[a] (Secretin, Boots)	c	1970		
Pancreozymin[b] (Pancreozymin, Boots)	c	—		

[a] International Nonproprietary Name.
[b] British Approved Name.
[c] Marketed; date unknown.

does not prevent relapse, nor apparently does it alter the long-term course of the disease. It possesses substantial mineralocorticoid-like side effects, which are, however, dose-dependent, predictable and manageable. Carbenoxolone is nevertheless the only presently marketed drug therapy that has been shown unequivocally to promote the healing of gastric ulcers. Deglycyrrhizinated licorice (Caved-S) has also been subjected to trials in both duodenal and gastric ulcer. Results to date have been mixed and in general are less satisfactory than those obtained with carbenoxolone; however, the side effects of deglycyrrhizinated licorice are less than those of carbenoxolone.

Carbenoxolone is clearly a useful drug and some of the studies proving its efficacy are models of experimental design in the field of clinical pharmacology.[78] In introducing a symposium on this compound, F. Avery Jones said,

> I believe the beneficial effect of carbenoxolone on the healing of gastric ulcers has been conclusively demonstrated. To say that it melts away ulcers would be an exaggeration! To say that it considerably facilitates the healing process and enables patients to be treated as outpatients and not in

hospital is a fair comment. . . . Is carbenoxolone a safe drug? For indiscriminate use without good supervision, the answer is no. But the same answer is true for almost every important drug we use in clinical medicine. Carbenoxolone has potential hazards and it is vitally important for the clinician to be aware of the possible risk of electrolyte disturbances and of hypertension. All side effects can be minimized or avoided when the drug is used with due care and discretion.[79]

In summarizing the same symposium, Watkinson said of carbenoxolone, "It has emerged as one of the most significant contributions to the treatment of gastric ulcer for fifty years and, although side effects limit its use, by selection of patients and the use of thiazide diuretics these side effects can largely be controlled. Its ability to prevent relapses and the complications of gastric ulcer has yet to be established."[80] The high acceptability of this agent to British experts has been documented.[81]

In the United States, the approach to this drug has been very different. Despite the fact that the drug had scarcely been investigated in the United States, Dr. Henry Simmons, then director of the Bureau of Drugs, FDA, testified at a meeting of the National Advisory Drug Committee that "American experts who know about the data [judged that] this drug should not be available in this country at this time. . . . Some studies show up to 30 percent side effects. . . ."[82] Although side effects do indeed limit the usefulness of carbenoxolone, it is still the only effective drug therapy available, and the consensus among experts who use this agent abroad is that benefits can be obtained when it is used in a way that reduces side effects to acceptable levels.[83]

If all agents for which "some studies showed a 30% incidence of side effects" were excluded from the market, few valuable drugs of any type would remain. It is, furthermore, revealing to note that at the time Dr. Simmons spoke carbenoxolone had been studied in fewer than twenty patients in the United States and the data from these patients had not by then been forwarded to the FDA. At that time, nearly 400 publications on carbenoxolone existed in the world's medical literature.

Metoclopramide (Maxolon) is an interesting compound which is structurally related to procainamide. It was first introduced as an antiemetic and is effective in this role[84] via a mechanism that may combine both central and peripheral sites of action. Subsequently, metoclopramide has been found to have striking effects on gastrointestinal motility in man. It accelerates gastric emptying by increasing peristaltic activity and relaxing the pylorus; transit time of substances through the stomach and small bowel is much reduced. This property has proved useful in radiology,[85] in the treatment of the flatulent dyspepsia syndromes,[86] and in emptying the stomach before anesthesia. It is not available in the U.S.

Pentagastrin (Peptavlon) is a synthetic gastrin-like pentapeptide. As a diagnostic agent for testing gastric secretion, pentagastrin is as effective as histamine and has fewer side effects.[87]

Discussion. The data presented show that for the decade up to the end of 1971 the overall British lead for mutually available drugs was, in terms of drug-years of prior availability, double that of the United States. In terms of exclusively available drugs, Britain had nearly four times as many as the United States. These data indicate that— at least in numerical terms—the United States has lagged considerably behind Britain in the introduction of new drugs.

Inspection of the record reveals that the international differences are larger and more distinct in some therapeutic categories than in others. The most clear-cut differences are apparent in the cardiovascular, diuretic, respiratory, and gastrointestinal areas. In these four areas, nearly all the exclusive drugs are available only in Britain, while introductions in the United States appear to have come almost to a halt despite the continuing introduction of new agents in these categories in Britain.

At the other end of the spectrum is cancer chemotherapy. There both countries have comparable numbers of exclusively available agents, but the range of those available is entirely different for each country and no outstandingly good or bad drugs can be discerned. Thus, in discussing the therapeutic implications of international differences, it is necessary to consider each therapeutic category separately.

It is worth remarking here that American physicians outside the Food and Drug Administration are likely to be uninformed about the toxicity of drugs available abroad but not in the United States. This problem was emphasized in a recent conference on adverse reaction reporting systems.[88] It is difficult to see how informed opinions on these drugs can at present be formulated by independent bodies, such as academic or professional groups, in the United States unless their information is obtained directly from abroad. There is much room for improvement in the availability of information to American physicians about comparative drug toxicity, both for drugs available here and for drugs available exclusively abroad.

In reviewing the literature pertaining to the drugs selected, a case emerges suggesting prima facie that over the past decade the United

States has been slow to introduce, and by the end of 1971 still lacked an appreciable number of, therapeutically useful drugs that had been available abroad for some years.

A rigorous consideration of overall benefit and loss involves more factors than those described here and needs to be dealt with in greater detail. If one accepts that the United States lags behind Britain in the introduction of new therapeutic drugs, two important questions follow: Are drugs that are unavailable in the United States but available in Britain *used* to an important extent in Britain? What are the therapeutic implications—both benefits and losses—of these differences? These matters will be considered in the next two chapters.

CHAPTER VIII

BRITISH USAGE AND AMERICAN AWARENESS OF SOME NEW DRUGS

As a first step toward determining the therapeutic significance of these international differences in drug availability, one needs to know whether and how the drugs that are exclusively available in Britain are actually being used there. If, for example, it were found that in certain therapeutic areas drugs exclusively available in Britain received widespread use there, then such areas would be identified as ones in which substantial differences might exist between British and American therapy as a result of differences in drug availability.

To determine overall British usage patterns, one could examine market research data to determine to what extent sales of newer agents erode the market for the older agents. Market research techniques are not, however, currently directed toward elucidating certain facts of greatest therapeutic interest: they do not show in enough detail what type of physician prescribes a particular drug, nor do they define the types of patients receiving it or the reasons for which the drug was chosen.

To obtain data on these points, we conducted a survey of British physicians at university teaching hospitals to determine how often experts in five selected therapeutic areas used certain new drugs available to them but not then to American physicians. We also compiled additional information to define in some detail the images British physicians had of the drugs they prescribed and of the relative performances, in their estimation, of the newer drugs versus older ones.

This chapter is an updated and condensed version of W. M. Wardell, "British Usage and American Awareness of Some New Therapeutic Drugs," *Clinical Pharmacology and Therapeutics*, vol. 14 (1973), pp. 1022-34. © 1973 by C. V. Mosby Company, St. Louis, Missouri.

For purposes of comparison, we also conducted a survey among physicians at an American university medical center to ascertain their knowledge of, and attitudes toward, these and other drugs that were in use abroad but not then available in the United States.

The results show that British experts make widespread use of certain new drugs, available exclusively to them, in the therapeutic areas surveyed. This has produced distinctly different therapeutic approaches to some common diseases in Britain and the United States. American physicians were found to be poorly informed about certain drugs highly regarded abroad but currently unavailable in the United States.

Methods

In the British survey, questionnaires were mailed in the period March through May 1972 to distributors at twenty British teaching hospitals and directed to physicians regarded as experts in five therapeutic areas: asthma, angina, hypertension, pyelonephritis, and gastric ulcer. The questionnaire presented a list of drugs, some exclusively available in Britain and the remainder mutually available in Britain and the United States. A pertinent clinical situation was described, and the recipient physician was asked to rate specified attributes of each drug—including frequency of choice, efficacy, and safety—as perceived by him in relation to that clinical situation.

The recipient was then asked to estimate in other ways the therapeutic impact of the drugs currently available only in Britain. One such estimate was to postulate what would result for his patients if those drugs were to be withdrawn from the market, forcing him to use alternative agents. This simulated the availability pattern in the United States, although the respondent was not informed of this fact nor that the drugs concerned were indeed available exclusively in Britain.

In the American survey, a questionnaire was sent during November and December 1971 to all 216 physicians associated with the Department of Medicine, University of Rochester School of Medicine and Dentistry, Rochester, New York. The questionnaire listed the following twelve drugs then available abroad but not in the United States: bethanidine (Esbatal), carbenoxolone (Biogastrone), clonidine (Catapres), debrisoquin (Declinax), cromolyn sodium (Intal), fusidic acid (Fucidin), orciprenaline (metaproterenol; Alupent), practolol (Eraldin), propanidid (Epontol), salbutamol (Ventolin), Slow-K, and trimethoprim-sulphamethoxazole (co-trimoxazole; Septra, Bactrim).

Each person was asked to check "yes" or "no" to the following questions about each drug:

Have you heard of this drug?
Could you describe its distinctive pharmacologic properties?
Could you describe its putative therapeutic advantages?
From your knowledge of it, would you want it available in the United States?

Further details of the methods and results of both surveys are given in the original publication.

Results of the British Survey

The results of this survey need to be interpreted cautiously since they consist of subjective estimates. It should be remembered, however, that for nearly all the questions asked in this study, no objective data yet exist. For example, the frequency of use of given drugs is not known for defined types of patients. Drug performance or efficacy has never been rigorously evaluated under conditions of actual use, as distinct from the conditions of controlled clinical trials. Comparative toxicity data are gradually becoming available from adverse reaction surveillance programs, but in most reporting schemes the data are ultimately derived—like the data in this study—from voluntary reports of physicians' impressions. For that matter, subjective impressions form the basis of most expert opinions. Furthermore, denominator values, that is, patient and drug exposure, are by no means universally available. Because of our paucity of objective knowledge about these matters, data of the type presented here will be important until superseded by more objective data.

The most secure information collected is the physician's indication of his own frequency of use of the various agents listed. The remaining data are softer than the data for frequency of use, but they can be used to define the images physicians have of the drugs they use in terms of efficacy, toxicity and certain other properties.

Asthma. Six bronchodilator drugs were listed: adrenaline (epinephrine), aminophylline, ephedrine, isoprenaline (isoproterenol), orciprenaline (metaproterenol), and salbutamol (albuterol). Recipients were first asked to rate each of four attributes of each drug on a scale of one to five, one being the most favorable and five being the least favorable score. The attributes were: frequency of choice, bronchodilator efficacy, incidence of severe side effects, and convenience for the patient. The ratings were made with respect to the

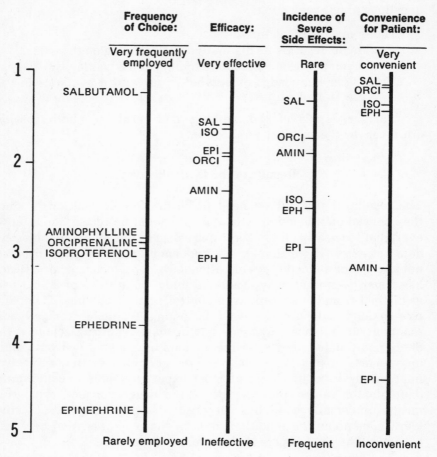

Figure 1

ASTHMA

responding physician's management, in his hospital outpatient clinic, of patients with chronic severe asthma who occasionally required steroids. (See Figure 1.)

Most of the interest in the results centers on the relative positions of the two agents then unavailable in the United States, namely, salbutamol and orciprenaline. It will be recalled that orciprenaline (metaproterenol) has subsequently been approved in the United States. Salbutamol was rated as by far the most frequently used agent. Salbutamol was also ranked first for the three other measures: efficacy, freedom from side effects, and convenience for the patient. Orciprenaline was used with less frequency, approximately the same as isoproterenol and aminophylline, and was ranked next to salbutamol in terms of convenience and freedom from side effects and close to epinephrine in efficacy.

In the second part of the questionnaire, the respondents evaluated the current impact of salbutamol and orciprenaline in asthma by predicting the effects that withdrawal of these agents and change to alternative therapy would have on the last ten patients they had treated with either agent.

It emerged—not unexpectedly in view of the known clinical pharmacology of these agents—that to some extent they can substitute for each other: withdrawal of both salbutamol and orciprenaline had considerably more predicted impact than the withdrawal of either one alone. These physicians estimated that only a third of the patients would be unaffected if salbutamol and orciprenaline were unavailable to them. Nearly half the patients would have worse control of bronchospasm and half would have more side effects. More than a quarter would find alternative therapy less convenient, and a fifth would comply less well with their therapeutic regimen. Twenty-eight percent of patients would require more steroids. Nineteen percent would have an impaired prognosis.

It is clear, therefore, that salbutamol has had a profound impact on the prescribing habits of the British experts and has displaced all other bronchodilator agents in the treatment of asthma in the type of patients described. Orciprenaline at present is used much less often than salbutamol, but would substitute for salbutamol if the latter were not available.

In terms of efficacy, side effects, and convenience, the images which physicians have of the clinical pharmacology of salbutamol and orciprenaline agree well with the known properties of these drugs. One cannot dissect out in retrospect the manner in which the prognosis of the 19 percent was thought to be impaired. This figure presumably includes those whose asthma becomes worse on alternative agents and those who suffer from the side effects—for example, cardiovascular—of alternative therapy.

Angina pectoris. Recipients were first asked to evaluate four anti-anginal drugs used in the treatment at their hospital outpatient clinic of patients with severe angina of effort. The agents were nitroglycerin, long-acting nitrates, the β-blockers, and prenylamine. They were asked to rate three attributes of each agent: frequency of choice, anti-anginal efficacy, and incidence of severe side effects. Beta-blockers and prenylamine are the two agents of interest here; prenylamine is not available in the United States, and the β-blockers

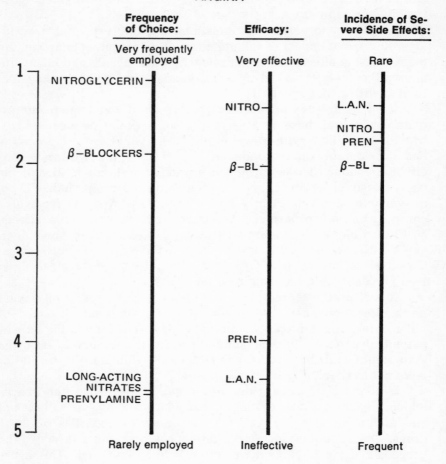

Figure 2
ANGINA

Frequency of Choice:	Efficacy:	Incidence of Severe Side Effects:
Very frequently employed	Very effective	Rare
NITROGLYCERIN —	NITRO —	L.A.N. —
		NITRO PREN —
β–BLOCKERS —	β–BL —	β–BL —
	PREN —	
LONG-ACTING NITRATES PRENYLAMINE	L.A.N. —	
Rarely employed	Ineffective	Frequent

were not then approved for the treatment of angina. In the responses, the β-blockers were the next most frequently chosen agents after nitroglycerin, and were regarded as next after nitroglycerin in effectiveness. On the other hand, they were regarded as having the most frequent side effects of the four agents listed, although this frequency was still relatively low. Prenylamine, by contrast, was the least frequently used of all these therapies and was regarded as only slightly more effective than long-acting nitrates. Its incidence of severe side effects was rated between those of nitroglycerin and the β-blockers. (See Figure 2.)

84

If the β-blockers were withdrawn and alternative therapy substituted, it was predicted that fewer than a third of patients currently treated with these agents would be unaffected. Two-thirds of them would have worse control of angina, half would find alternative therapy less convenient, one-quarter would have more side effects, in one-quarter there would be less compliance with the regimen, and in a fifth there would be an impaired prognosis.

The β-blockers have clearly made a large impact in the treatment of angina. The comments in response to this questionnaire indicated that the β-blockers were generally reserved for those patients in whom nitroglycerin had failed. This selection presumably accounts for the strikingly high proportion of patients expected to be adversely affected if the β-blockers were withdrawn. The question of impaired prognosis was a problematic one. Many of the respondents correctly indicated that the influence of all the agents listed on the prognosis of angina was unknown. Those who did respond with an estimate frequently gave a reason, usually the anti-arrhythmic action of the β-blockers.

Hypertension. Recipients were first asked to rate eight antihypertensive drugs in the management of moderately severe hypertensive patients attending the recipient's hospital outpatient clinic. The drugs were methyldopa, diuretics, guanethidine, reserpine, hydralazine, bethanidine, clonidine, and the β-blockers. They were asked to rate each agent in three respects: frequency of choice, hypotensive efficacy, and incidence of severe side effects. The three agents of special interest are bethanidine and clonidine, which are not available in the United States, and the β-blockers, which are not approved for the management of hypertension in this country. (See Figure 3.)

It was found that by far the most frequently chosen agents were diuretics and methyldopa. Then there were three drugs—the β-blockers, bethanidine, and guanethidine—that were used with lower but approximately equal frequency. Clonidine came after these agents, and at the bottom of the list was hydralazine, preceded by reserpine.

The image of bethanidine was that it was slightly less effective than the pharmacologically similar compound, guanethidine, but had fewer side effects; conversely, it was more effective than methyldopa but had more side effects.

The β-blocking drugs were rated as being slightly less effective than the diuretics but more effective than reserpine or hydralazine. On the other hand, the incidence of severe side effects produced by

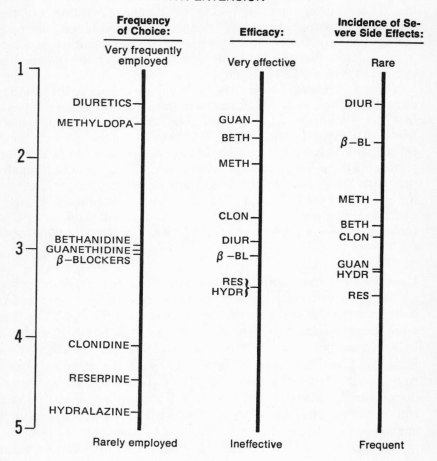

Figure 3

HYPERTENSION

Frequency of Choice:	Efficacy:	Incidence of Severe Side Effects:

Very frequently employed — Very effective — Rare

1 —

DIURETICS —
METHYLDOPA —

GUAN —
BETH —
METH —

DIUR —
β—BL —

2 —

CLON —
DIUR —
β—BL —

METH —
BETH —
CLON —

3 —
BETHANIDINE
GUANETHIDINE
β—BLOCKERS

RES }
HYDR }

GUAN
HYDR

RES —

4 —
CLONIDINE —

RESERPINE —

HYDRALAZINE —

5 —

Rarely employed — Ineffective — Frequent

the β-blockers was felt to be more frequent than with the diuretics but less than with methyldopa.

Clonidine was seldom chosen, although it was chosen more frequently than reserpine. It was regarded as being between diuretics and methyldopa in effectiveness, and between methyldopa and guanethidine in producing severe side effects.

It was felt that withdrawal of the β-blockers, bethanidine and clonidine, would be of importance in more than half the patients in whom any of the three were being used: nearly half of these patients would have worse control of hypertension, nearly half would have more side effects, approximately one-third of the patients would show less compliance with the regimen, and one-third would have an impaired prognosis.

Although the agents exclusively available in Britain are not the agents of first choice there, bethanidine and the β-blockers have made a moderate impact on prescribing patterns in hypertension, being used in this situation with a frequency approximately equal to that of guanethidine. The low frequency of use of clonidine probably reflects another variable influencing a drug's success, that is, the length of time for which it has been available. Clonidine was approved for use in the United Kingdom only a few months before this questionnaire was circulated. Presumably a new agent does not become established overnight; if this same survey were to be repeated at different times, the relative positions of the agents would change, reflecting the advent of new therapy and all the factors and pressures accompanying it which influence a physician's decision to prescribe.

The estimates of efficacy and side effects of all these antihypertensive agents are consistent with their known properties. Estimates of noncompliance and of impaired prognosis are probably more valid in hypertension than in any of the other therapeutic categories of this study. In the absence of data to the contrary, it is reasonable to assume that the presence of more side effects would render patients on alternate agents less likely to comply with those therapeutic regimens and that impaired control of blood pressure due to lack of compliance leads to an impaired prognosis.

Gastric ulcer. The physicians were first asked to evaluate seven therapeutic entities in the treatment of gastric ulcer: antacids, anticholinergic drugs, diet, sedatives, bed rest, surgery (without trial of nonsurgical regimens), and carbenoxolone. Of the therapies listed, only the last three have been shown to have efficacy, and carbenoxolone is the one that is not available in the United States. The recipients were asked to rate these agents with respect to the management of patients seen at the recipient's hospital outpatient clinic with newly diagnosed benign gastric ulcers having symptoms of three months' duration. They were asked to rate four attributes of each therapy: frequency of choice, success rate in promoting healing, incidence of severe side effects, and convenience for the patient. (See Figure 4.)

In terms of efficacy, carbenoxolone appeared high on the list, being ranked next in effectiveness to surgery and more effective than bed rest. All other therapies were ranked very low.

Figure 4

GASTRIC ULCER

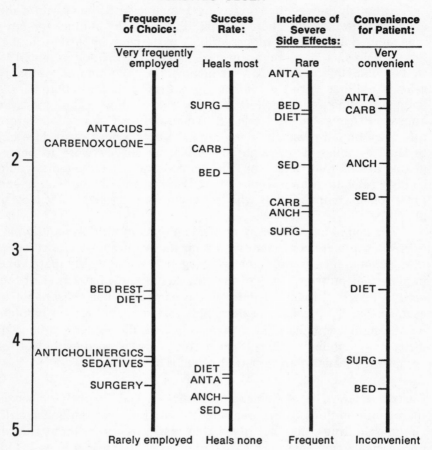

In terms of frequency of choice, carbenoxolone was by far the most frequently employed of the three active therapies. Carbenoxolone was, indeed, employed nearly as often as antacid therapy. Bed rest was much less frequently employed, while surgery as initial therapy was used least often.

The perceived incidence of severe side effects with carbenoxolone was appreciable but not excessive, being ranked between those of sedatives and anticholinergic agents.

In terms of convenience for the patient, carbenoxolone was ranked close to antacids, and both of these were ranked much higher than any of the other therapies.

If carbenoxolone were withdrawn, necessitating alternative therapy, it was estimated that fewer than one-third of patients currently receiving carbenoxolone would be unaffected. More than half would have slower healing of the ulcer, and a fifth would have no healing at all. One-third would need to be hospitalized, and more than one-quarter would need prolonged bed rest at home. It was estimated that one-fifth of the patients treated with carbenoxolone were being spared surgery.

Thus, in terms of efficacy, the responding physicians made a clear distinction between the three therapies listed that have been proved to promote healing (surgery, bed rest, and carbenoxolone) and the other therapies, which are of only symptomatic value. Carbenoxolone was the most frequently used of all the effective therapies and has had a major impact on the therapeutic approach of these British experts. Its perceived efficacy and convenience for the patient clearly outweighed its appreciable incidence of side effects. The small proportion of patients in whom it was estimated that carbenoxolone was preventing surgery is in keeping with the currently known properties of this compound; although its efficacy in accelerating the healing of a gastric ulcer is now undisputed, it has not been clearly shown to prevent relapse or to alter the natural history of the disease or the ultimate need for surgery. In view of the known toxicity of carbenoxolone, it was of interest to see that those who are using it do not rate the side effects as too severe. This may be a reflection of the fact that although the mineralocorticoid side effects of this agent are frequently experienced, they are predictable, dose-dependent, and familiar, and can be anticipated or corrected.

Pyelonephritis. Recipients were first asked to evaluate ten antibacterial agents in the management of pyelonephritis. The drugs were ampicillin, carbenicillin, the cephalosporins, chloramphenicol, gentamicin, nalidixic acid, co-trimoxazole, nitrofurantoin, the sulfonamides, and the tetracyclines. Recipients were asked to base their responses on their management of a patient with chronic pyelonephritis who appeared at their outpatient clinic with an acute, severe flare-up. Urinary culture and sensitivity results were assumed to be available. The following properties of each agent were rated: current prevalence of resistant organisms, frequency of choice (assuming the organism is sensitive), efficacy in eradicating a sensitive organism when used in full dosage, and incidence of side effects necessitating change in therapy. The agent which was not then available in the United States, and upon which most attention in this section is focused, is co-trimoxazole (Septra, Burroughs Wellcome and Bactrim,

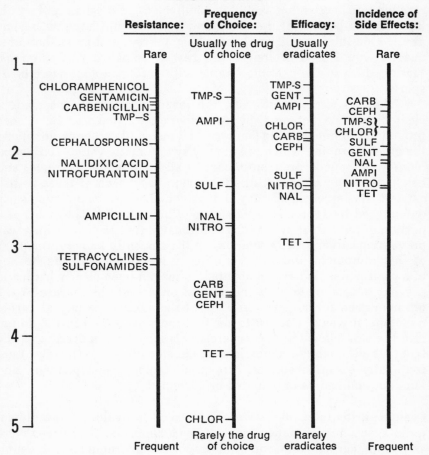

Figure 5

PYELONEPHRITIS

Roche), the properties of which were discussed earlier. It can be seen that in terms of rarity of resistant organisms, co-trimoxazole was then ranked among the best: close to gentamicin, superior to the cephalosporins, and considerably better than ampicillin. Where an organism was sensitive to it, co-trimoxazole was, moreover, regarded as the drug of choice, ahead of ampicillin and very much ahead of the sulfonamides alone. In terms of efficacy, co-trimoxazole was again the agent rated first, ahead of gentamicin and ampicillin. The incidence of side effects with co-trimoxazole necessitating a change of therapy was relatively low, being ranked less than with ampicillin and gentamicin and similar to the incidence with the sulfonamides alone. (See Figure 5.)

If co-trimoxazole had not been available, forcing the use of alternative therapy, it was predicted that somewhat more than half the patients would experience no difference. In 15 percent there would be a necessity for parenteral therapy. In 22 percent of the patients the organism would be insensitive to alternative agents, and in 27 percent there would be less prospect of eradicating the organism. However, there would be an increased risk of further renal impairment in only 7 percent. In 22 percent there would be a greater likelihood of adverse drug reactions. It was estimated that 11 percent of the patients would need admission to the hospital.

Thus, co-trimoxazole has had an impressive impact on prescribing patterns in pyelonephritis, as seen from its rating as the agent of first choice in the situation described, even when the microorganism is sensitive to other agents, such as ampicillin, as well.

Results of the Rochester Survey

The average respondent signified that he had heard of only 1.6 of the twelve drugs listed in the questionnaire, that he knew either the distinctive pharmacologic features, the putative therapeutic advantages, or both of 0.9 drugs, and that he would like to have 0.7 of this 0.9 available to him in the United States.

The subsequent analysis was confined to those respondents whom we could regard as experts in each therapeutic area. For this purpose, replies from physicians identifiable with specific subspecialty departments, that is, above the house-staff level, were used.

In general, these physicians had a low level of awareness of the drugs listed. Even when analysis is stratified by the specialist groups to whom the drugs would be of greatest relevance, the results still show that most of these drugs are essentially unknown in the United States. This includes even those that are, as shown in the British survey, in very wide use abroad and for which substantial documentation is available.[2] Only six out of forty-five physicians in the relevant specialties (in this case, pulmonary medicine, allergy, cardiology and internal medicine) had heard of salbutamol; six out of forty had heard of bethanidine; none out of forty-seven (indeed, none of the 134 respondents who had practiced only within the United States) had heard of Slow-K; eight out of twenty-one had heard of carbenoxolone; and seven out of thirty-three had heard of co-trimoxazole. There were only two drugs for which the level of awareness exceeded 50 percent of the specialists concerned: twenty-five of thirty-nine had heard of practolol, and seventeen of twenty-four had heard of cromolyn sodium. This latter figure was presumably due to the fact that cromolyn sodium had recently undergone a clinical trial in the hospital.

In general, the number of respondents who knew something about a drug, either its distinctive pharmacological properties or putative therapeutic advantages, was substantially less than the number who had heard of the drug. However, when a respondent signified that he did know about a drug's properties, he usually expressed the desire to have it available to him in the United States. Thus, all nineteen respondents who signified that they knew of the properties of practolol also wished to have it available in the United States. The corresponding figures for some of the other drugs were fourteen out of fourteen for cromolyn sodium, four out of five for clonidine and for salbutamol, and five out of six for carbenoxolone. On the other hand, some drugs were not as highly desired. One out of three respondents wanted to have bethanidine, and two out of four wanted to have co-trimoxazole; these numbers are obviously small and perhaps do not reflect differences in opinion as dramatically as the percentages might indicate.

Conclusions

In the therapeutic areas surveyed and for the conditions described, certain drugs then unavailable in the United States had made a great impact on the prescribing habits of British experts. The therapy chosen by physicians at British teaching hospitals for the patients described was substantially different from that which could at that time be prescribed by American physicians. This therapy includes the β-blockers in angina, salbutamol in asthma, co-trimoxazole in pyelonephritis, carbenoxolone in gastric ulcer, and to a lesser but still important degree, the β-blockers and bethanidine in hypertension. These drugs have been available abroad for periods ranging from six years in the case of salbutamol to a decade in the case of carbenoxolone and of bethanidine.

If Rochester physicians are representative, the level of knowledge which American physicians have of these drugs is very low, even among experts in the appropriate specialties. It is, moreover, worthy of note that those few American physicians who were aware of a drug's properties usually signified a desire to have the drug available in the United States.

CHAPTER IX

THERAPEUTIC CONSEQUENCES OF THE DRUG LAG

In the previous two chapters we examined some of the benefits and losses that have accrued to Britain and the United States as a result of their different approaches to the introduction of new drugs in certain therapeutic areas. In the present chapter, we examine the wider therapeutic implications of these international differences in approach: compared with the United States, does Britain benefit from having more, or more effective, drugs available? Or does Britain suffer because the newer drugs available there are less effective or more toxic than those mutually available? In wider terms, what is the overall value to society of the whole process of drug innovation?

The Measurement of Therapeutic Impact

To measure the total medical impact of a new therapeutic drug in a society, one would ideally need to perform an experiment. For example, the drug could be introduced into certain communities and withheld from other comparable ones in a randomized, controlled manner. Objective data could then be collected on the therapeutic outcome of relevant diseases in the control versus the test communities, and these could be weighed against the total drug toxicity recorded under the same conditions of use. Simultaneously, measurements could be made of the extent to which the new drug replaced older treatments. The therapeutic outcome—beneficial or toxic—could be assigned in each case to the treatment used. If all the rele-

---

This chapter is an updated and condensed version of W. M. Wardell, "Therapeutic Implications of the Drug Lag," *Clinical Pharmacology and Therapeutics*, vol. 15 (1974), pp. 73-96. © 1973 by C. V. Mosby Company, St. Louis, Missouri.

vant data were obtained, then the actual therapeutic impact of that drug could be defined.

This experimental approach has never been attempted, although technically it would be possible with the record-linkage schemes now operating in some countries. Since such comprehensive data are not available, we need to examine other approaches to assessing the therapeutic impact of contemporary drugs.

One logical approach is to construct a balance sheet of the currently measurable benefits and losses stemming from introduction of a drug. Benefit as a therapeutic concept involving a whole society's response to a drug has not yet been well defined or measured. This lack is illustrated by the literature involving therapeutic trials. That which deals with the controlled clinical trials prescribed by the FDA for Phases II and III of the IND procedure describes the results obtained when drugs are administered under defined and controlled conditions to specific types of patients. The larger scale, often uncontrolled, postmarketing trials (Phase IV) provide wider experience of treated disease, but in a manner whereby the therapeutic contribution of the drug under study may be unmeasurable. None of the current methods of drug evaluation are designed to measure the total impact of the drug under conditions of actual use—that is, when given in an unmonitored way to undefined patients. In short, therapeutic trials do not tell us how the drug actually performs in practice.

At best then, therapeutic trials can measure only the potential benefit and harm available from a drug, not the benefit and harm actually realized in the community. Other kinds of data must be obtained to build a complete picture.

Even if these difficulties in extrapolation were not present, the primary drug literature has other pitfalls which prove fatal. One could diligently and, with computer assistance, exhaustively search the literature, evaluate positive versus negative reports, and come to an "impartial" conclusion about a drug. However, the impartiality of such a conclusion is illusory. It is biased to an unknown extent by the many selection processes—academic, industrial, personal and editorial—which operate before a report of any scientific study can reach the literature. The value of impartial reviews of the drug literature is therefore open to question.[1]

Risk associated with new drugs is somewhat easier to assess because a different kind of methodology has been developed. Over the past decade, drug adverse reaction surveillance programs have been developed using a variety of different approaches. All such programs have limitations stemming from the quality of the data and their mode of acquisition. Nevertheless, some of these programs have the ability to estimate a drug's total harm to the community and the comparative toxicity of different drugs. These toxicity data are obviously much more germane to the task of measuring the impact of drugs than the type of data available for describing drug benefits.

In addition to surveillance data, there is an extensive case-report literature on adverse drug reactions. While this suffers from the same defects as case report data for describing benefit, it does help to define in more detail the nature of the toxicity revealed by surveillance programs.

From the foregoing consideration of medical risk and benefit measurement an important fact emerges. A situation has arisen in which we now have methodology available which, while defective, is being used to estimate the total harm of drugs to the community; but we have no comparable methodology available for measuring the total benefit of drugs to the community. We are therefore poorly equipped to undertake the sophisticated risk-benefit analyses required for optimal drug prescribing, since the known hazards of a drug tend to overshadow its unknown benefits. This imbalance affects therapeutic decisions at all levels, from the physician who prescribes drugs for patients to the regulatory agency that anticipates the total impact of drugs on the community and sets physicians' prescribing boundaries accordingly.

So far we have viewed the measurement of therapeutic impact in medical terms. An alternative approach is economic. One example of this is "Cost Analysis of Selected Diseases," a study by Arthur D. Little, Inc.[2] Another, more comprehensive study that is closely relevant to the drug lag is that of Peltzman.[3] In these approaches, epidemiological and actuarial data on disease trends and outcomes were analyzed. The costs of mortality and morbidity were computed from loss of earnings and costs of treatment. By choosing appropriate disease situations and by making assumptions about the role of drug therapy in changing the outcome of diseases, the economic benefits and costs of therapy could be estimated. Peltzman considered a number of other issues also, including the costs to society of delaying the introduction of successful drug therapies. Some results of these economic studies have already been discussed.

With medical approaches in mind, we can now examine the feasibility of making a risk-benefit analysis of the drug lag. For a drug mutually available in the United States and Britain, the assessment is relatively straightforward. The fact that a drug has received marketing approval in both countries denotes that, in the opinion of both their regulatory agencies, the drug's therapeutic benefits outweigh its risks. Provided that the drug has not subsequently been withdrawn for toxicity reasons, the country which introduced that drug first can be considered to have gained from its promptness. Although the existence of this advantage is clear, its size and importance are more difficult to assess. The most obvious cases are those of drugs that are the first, only, or currently most important members of new pharmacologic classes. The potential therapeutic contribution of such agents can usually be judged from the results of clinical trials in which that agent is compared with the previously available therapy; however, the interpretation, for this purpose, of clinical trial results requires some comment.

When clinical trials are arranged to compare two active therapies, it is rare, with current techniques, to demonstrate large or significant differences in efficacy between active drugs. Where a difference has been shown, it usually exists for only one or two dose levels. Dose-effect curves are seldom adequately defined in human studies, so that reported differences are often uninterpretable.

Failure to show a difference in efficacy between a new drug and an older one should not be taken to mean that the newer compound cannot be a worthwhile advance, even if the statistical power of the study, which is rarely calculated, is adequate. First, each drug's efficacy may be exerted on a different segment of the population; if both drugs were available, the proportion of patients treatable might be much higher than if either drug were available alone. By the same argument, a drug that is on average less effective and more toxic than existing therapy may still be highly desirable for some segments of the population. Our current simplistic statistical concepts of efficacy and safety usually fail to take this into account. Second, it is common to find that the spectrum of side effects differs for each agent, or that the pharmacokinetics are different enough to require different dosage regimens for each drug. Third, in the actual treatment of many types of conditions, a patient may receive several drugs in turn on a trial-and-error basis until the one that is best for his needs is determined empirically. These realities of therapeutics for individual patients are generally ignored in the current requirements for evidence of drug efficacy. All these factors can be crucial for tailoring therapy to an individual patient to achieve maximal efficacy, safety, comfort, convenience, and compliance with the therapeutic regimen. To achieve these goals it is desirable to have alternative therapies from which to choose.

The benefits of leads in the introduction of subsequent members of a pharmacologic class, pejoratively called "me-too" drugs, are usually of a smaller degree, but the nature of the evidence is in some ways easier to assess. Clinical trials of newer members of a series are frequently arranged to test the new member against the initial one. Here the same arguments apply: even if one cannot discriminate between members of a series in terms of average efficacy, the availability of alternatives means that there is greater scope for tailoring therapy to an individual patient than if no choice were possible.

For drugs that are exclusively available in one country, the analysis is potentially more complex, since these drugs may not have satisfied the other country's criteria for efficacy and safety. However, assessing the safety of drugs exclusively available in Britain is easier than assessing the safety of those available exclusively in the United States. This is because of the availability of summarized data from adverse reaction surveillance programs in Britain and some other countries; comparable summaries of the American experience are not available. The British data, while not published, can be obtained in the form of an extensive (600-page) printed summary from the British Committee on Safety of Medicines. This summary has been used as part of the evidence in examining the toxicity patterns of drugs discussed in this paper. Such data on human toxicity should be more helpful than American studies on animals.

In examining the balance sheet for individual therapeutic categories (Chapter VII), it was shown that, in many therapeutic areas, useful and even uniquely effective or safe drugs have been introduced in Britain substantially earlier than in the United States, and at any given time the United States lacks a number of such drugs. While the areas most affected are those of cardiovascular, diuretic, respiratory, antibacterial and gastrointestinal therapy, some effect can be discerned in most areas surveyed, at the very least in terms of delayed introduction in the United States.

One should next examine whether Britain has suffered from the introduction of drugs that are less effective than older agents or are ineffective. It is difficult to find clear-cut examples of harm arising from this cause. First, as discussed earlier, a drug that has some activity generally has enough distinguishing features to offer special advantages to certain patients. Second, to prove that a drug has no activity involves trying to prove the null hypothesis and seems an exercise not worth attempting. Since the individual patient may have been treated with a series of agents to find the most suitable one, it is as difficult to disprove that some patients have benefited from drugs that are on average unimpressive as it is to prove that others have suffered. Furthermore, it can be assumed that recent judgments in the United Kingdom about drug approvals are based on reasonable evidence of therapeutic activity.

Despite these considerations, one should ask whether some harm has resulted from the introduction of new drugs that are less effective than the existing ones and whether Britain has suffered more such harm than the United States—if only because the total number of new drugs introduced into Britain was greater. The real questions are, what is the size of the total problem in both countries due to relatively ineffective drugs, and what fraction of this is due to those exclusively available in Britain? There are no data available to answer these questions comprehensively. However, it should be noted that the total number of all new drugs introduced exclusively into Britain over the decade was greatly outweighed by the number of older drugs and combinations already available in the United States which, on the available evidence, were subsequently rated as "ineffective" in the U.S. drug efficacy study. Of 369 products so rated in the United States, only 90 identical or closely similar products were available in Britain. This fact, combined with the opportunity to try various drugs in specific cases, suggests that inefficacious drugs are unlikely to have made a disproportionate—or even an appreciable—impact on British therapeutics.

Since beneficial new drugs are introduced more quickly and in greater numbers in Britain, one may ask whether that country suffers from more new drug toxicity than the United States. The answer is obviously yes, since a drug's toxicity—like its benefits—will only occur where the drug is actually being used, and many more new drugs were introduced into Britain. This question is not, however, the most relevant one. What we really need to know is, first, the total drug toxicity occurring in each country; second, how serious the problem of new drug toxicity is in comparison with that total; third, whether Britain shows any obvious examples of toxicity due to drugs which were introduced there under the current regulatory system, but which have been excluded from the United States; and fourth, whether the toxicity seen with newer drugs is counterbalanced by greater therapeutic benefit.

The first of these questions cannot be answered because drug surveillance schemes are not yet comprehensive and uniform enough to enable one to compare international incidence figures. Nevertheless, a comparison of the scope and performance of the surveillance systems that currently exist in Britain and the United States is itself illuminating. In terms of voluntary spontaneous reporting rates, the data base of the British scheme is substantially larger than the American one. Over the four-year period to the end of 1971, the British voluntary reporting rate was nearly ten times that of the United States on a per capita basis.[4] American voluntary reporting of drug toxicity is the lowest, or nearly so, of all countries reporting to the WHO monitoring project; the total number of reports from the whole of the United States for 1971 was one-quarter the number reported from Canada.[5] In contrast to the British policy, summaries of the American adverse experience have never been published, nor have the data been made available for independent research or study. The British system includes feedback from the monitor to the reporting physician, follow-up of selected reactions by a staff of eighty part-time physicians throughout the country, and facilities for intensive monitoring after release of any drug about which there is special concern.[6] Furthermore, the British system is well regarded in international terms: the FDA warnings in 1966 and 1969 regarding the thromboembolic risk with oral contraceptives were based solely on British or British-Scandinavian studies; no definitive American studies were available at the time.[7] Thus, the British system of postmarketing surveillance is much better geared than the American system to detecting hazards from new drugs at the point when they assume the greatest importance.

Despite these advantages, there has been at least one instance in which the British surveillance system has not been adequate. This was the epidemic of asthma deaths which occurred in the 1960s. In that instance, it has been pointed out that time and lives could have been saved if an Australian warning, issued three years earlier, had been given greater weight at the time.[8] Two points should, however, be noted about the asthma mortality. First, it was not associated with a new drug, nor even with a new dose form of an older drug. Even the Stolley hypothesis, which has never been proposed by its author as the sole explanation, implicates a dose form, introduced years earlier, of the old established drug isoproterenol.[9] No application was made to market this strength of isoproterenol in the United States. Second, since all hypotheses of the epidemic's cause involve excessive use of the drug, this is precisely the type of adverse reaction that could not be reliably detected and intercepted in the premarketing phase.

The second question, concerning the contribution of new drugs to total drug toxicity, can be answered conclusively. We shall concentrate mainly on those adverse reactions severe enough to cause death.

The most relevant published British data consist of a series of 100 randomly chosen spontaneous adverse drug reaction reports that were followed up in a research project to determine the accuracy of assumptions concerning the causal role of specific drugs.[10] In this series, there were fourteen fatalities ultimately judged to be probably due to the drugs named; in all fourteen cases, the drug had been available in Britain for at least ten years and was also available in the United States. There were in addition seventeen serious but nonfatal reactions in which a specific causal drug was identified. Only four of these involved drugs which are not available in the United States, and in each case the nearest American equivalent is well known to be capable of producing identical toxicity.

Further relevant data are available from the New Zealand Committee on Adverse Drug Reactions. The New Zealand data are published annually [11] and more details were obtained from that committee. The pattern of introduction of new drugs in New Zealand closely resembles that of Britain rather than the United States, and New Zealand's rate of voluntary reporting of adverse drug reactions, as compiled by the WHO monitoring project, is the highest of all reporting countries: on a per capita basis, the reporting rate is more than double that of Britain, and twenty times that of the United States.[12]

Over the four-year period ending in March 1972, 2,175 reports of adverse drug reactions were received, of which 93 were fatal.[13] With the proviso that we are dealing entirely with drugs listed as being associated with each fatality, and not with proved causality, the 93 fatalities may be analyzed as follows:

Twenty-four percent of the patients who died had been taking a new drug, defined here as a drug marketed in New Zealand since 1968 or not available in the United States. However, most of these patients had also been taking another, older drug well known to be a cause of the reaction concerned, for example, phenylbutazone in a case of aplastic anemia. Excluding such cases, we find only 6.5 percent of the deaths were associated with new drugs without other possible causes being present.

Most of the fatalities were associated with well-known properties of older drugs. Where a known or likely association could be derived from inspection of the drugs listed and the fatal reaction produced, the drug in question had, in over 90 percent of the cases, been available for more than five years and in nearly half the cases for more than ten years.

Adverse reactions to newer drugs are likely to be reported more faithfully than reactions to older drugs: not only are patients and physicians more suspicious of new drugs, but the monitoring system specifically exhorts doctors to report all adverse experience with new drugs. For these reasons, percentages of deaths associated with new drugs are almost certainly overestimates. It is clear from these data that the bulk of the worst drug toxicity recognized at present is due, not to unsuspected reactions to new or unusual drugs, but to well-recognized and familiar reactions to old established drugs.

Similar conclusions emerge from two North American studies. Shapiro et al. recorded twenty-seven iatrogenic deaths among more than 6,000 consecutive medical inpatients.[14] Only two of the twenty-seven deaths were associated with new or recent drugs. Ogilvie and Ruedy, in a similar study of medical inpatients, found that more than half the adverse reactions were caused by drugs that had been in use for over thirty years, while most of the remainder were due to drugs that had been in use for more than ten years. They observed that "it cannot be said that the high incidence of reactions was due to new drugs with which the medical profession has had little experience."[15]

The third question, as to whether toxic drugs have been introduced into Britain but excluded from the United States during the current regulatory era, can be approached in two ways. The first is to examine those drugs which became exclusively available in Britain and which were later withdrawn or restricted there for toxicity reasons. Ignoring any benefits conferred by these drugs, we may regard them as cases in which the United States entirely escaped toxicity incurred in the process of drug development and marketing in Britain. The toxicity of two of these drugs, benziodarone and ibufenac, has been fully reviewed previously;[16] in numerical terms, they contributed negligibly to total drug toxicity.[17] While toxic effects on individual patients are to be regretted, credit is due to the monitoring system in Britain for the detection of these effects at such an early stage. Furthermore, one should not overlook the fact that older alternative agents may themselves possess considerable toxicity. Arthritic patients, given the option, might justifiably have preferred the risk of acquiring reversible hepatic disease with ibufenac to the smaller but catastrophic hazard of irreversible aplastic anemia with phenylbutazone. The only other example which we have been able to identify was the long-established disinfectant dequalinium which, when extended to a new application as a diaper disinfectant, caused dermal ulceration. Again, while toxicity in this situation outweighed the advantages it conferred, in the context of the whole process of drug development and use, the actual damage produced (according to data made available to the authors) was small both in extent and degree.

The second approach to the examination of drugs excluded for toxicity reasons from the United States but available in Britain is offered by a recent statement made by the FDA before the Subcommittee on Monopoly of the Senate Select Committee on Small Business.[18] Exhibit 5 of that statement lists twenty-six drugs for which clinical evaluation was limited, having been discontinued by the manufacturer or terminated by the FDA for safety reasons in the United States, but which were on the market in other countries despite these problems. The drugs were not identified by name in Exhibit 5, but their properties and toxicity were outlined. We have obtained from the FDA the names of twelve of these drugs, which could be disclosed under the current interpretation of the Freedom of Information Act, and there are two others which can be positively identified from internal evidence in the statement. These fourteen drugs will now be considered.

Nine had been introduced into Britain during the period covered by the present study (1962–71). The toxicity of four of these (guanoxan, ibufenac, practolol and oxprenolol) has already been discussed.

Nifuratel (Magmilor) is an agent with anti-trichomonal and antifungal activity. Its putative toxicity was described in Exhibit 5 as "similar to compounds shown to be carcinogenic [in animals]." Presumably this refers to a structural similarity, raising again the difficult problem of guilt by structural association which characterizes the debate over the newer β-blockers. It must be acknowledged that the best course of action concerning such compounds is not yet known, and different interpretations are tenable. Nevertheless, the logic of the present example is, at best, tenuous. While the identity of the "similar compounds" referred to is not clear, the obvious candidate is metronidazole, the prototype drug and still the most extensively used agent in the field of anti-trichomonal therapy in all countries. Metronidazole produces lung tumors and malignant lymphomas in mice.[19] It could be argued that if animal carcinogenicity is a reason for excluding a compound from the market, it would be more logical to exclude metronidazole than nifuratel, since the latter has so far been shown only to resemble compounds shown to be carcinogenic in animals, while the former actually is carcinogenic.

Two of the remaining drugs were listed as discontinued or terminated because of animal toxicity: verapamil (Cordilox) caused "cataracts—dogs" and bromhexine (Bisolvon) caused "convulsions—dogs, rats" and "increased incidence of mammary tumors and possibility of cataracts—rats."[20] The remaining two compounds listed in Exhibit 5 and available in Britain are opipramol (Insidon) and trifluperidol (Triperidol). In the case of these two agents, human toxicity was cited. The nature of these human side effects listed in Exhibit 5 was, however, precisely that of alternative agents in their general class of psychotropic drugs.

Two important types of data are needed to clarify the implications of these latter disclosures: utilization figures and surveillance data relating to the drugs in Britain. It does not appear that utilization of any of these drugs was extensive in relation to other agents in the same therapeutic classes. Sales of bromhexine, opipramol, and trifluperidol were too small to be listed separately in a British market research summary for 1972, while verapamil sales accounted for only 1.9 percent of the market for anti-anginal agents.[21] Surveillance and other data did not reveal excessively distinctive or unexpected adverse-reaction patterns.

While it does not appear from the evidence available that an excessive hazard exists with these drugs, either intrinsically or with the ways they are used in Britain, this should not be taken to exonerate any of the drugs listed in Exhibit 5. The FDA's testimony published in that document should stimulate careful scrutiny, by authorities in those countries where they are available, of all the drugs listed. Nevertheless, the data revealed so far in support of the exclusion of these drugs from the American market do not in themselves prove that this exclusion is beneficial to the American patient, or that other countries have suffered from the introduction of these drugs.

From this discussion of drug toxicity it can be seen that if one wishes to reduce the burden of drug toxicity in the community, new drugs are not the place to start. *Efforts would be better directed to optimizing the use of all hazardous drugs, rather than to restricting the availability of newer agents, which contribute so minimally to the problem.* Any preventable drug toxicity must clearly be avoided, but in the real world the only way to abolish it entirely would be to abolish all drugs and thus forego their benefits entirely. Since most serious drug toxicity can be shown to stem from older, well established drugs, there appears to be no foundation for the customary belief that new drugs represent the greatest hazard. One could indeed advance a plausible case for the opposite view: because both physicians and their patients now tend to be wary of new drugs, it is entirely possible that the extra caution surrounding their use could make them safer in practice than older, more familiar alternatives.

Are there any other ways in which either country could have gained or lost from its respective approach toward the introduction of new drugs? It has been argued by some that the introduction of more drugs is confusing to the physician. From the data compiled in this study, a plausible case along these lines could be made only for the field of psychotropic drugs. Moreover, the availability of more new drugs in the United Kingdom is far outweighed by the availability of many more forms of older drugs (brands and combinations) in the United States: nearly 2,500 items are listed for prescription in the British MIMS,[22] while close to 6,700 separate products were listed in the 1972 edition of the American *Physicians' Desk Reference*.[23]

It is hard to find any clear advantages accruing to American physicians from having a smaller range of distinct chemical entities from which to choose. As already pointed out, demonstrable differences in overall efficacy among active drugs are less common than differences in response among patients and in the nature of side effects. A wide selection of effective agents is therefore desirable in order that therapy may be tailored to the individual patient. We may not always know how to select patients to make optimal use of the choice of drugs available, but this argues for more knowledge and perseverance, rather than for fewer drugs.

In economic terms, the conclusion of the most important study of that aspect to date is disturbing. Peltzman estimated that the effect of the 1962 amendments to the Food, Drug and Cosmetic Act has been to cost the American consumer at least $250 to $350 million annually, or about 6 percent of total drug sales.[24] Peltzman's argument was in absolute terms. Since regulation of the drug development process has become more rigorous in Britain also since 1962, some losses may have been incurred there as well. But Peltzman dealt with areas in which, as shown in the present study, the British situation seems to compare favorably with that of the United States. Thus, the British patient has probably gained economically in comparison with his American counterpart.

In addition to economic factors, one should consider the influence of drug regulatory policies on the existence and innovative output of the research-based pharmaceutical industry, which has been responsible for nearly all new therapeutic drug discoveries.

In Chapter V, we pointed out the steep rise that has occurred over the past decade in the cost of developing a new single drug entity in the United States and the inhibitory effect that this may be having on the industry's willingness to explore new areas where remuneration may not be clearly foreseeable. The time required for a drug to undergo the required testing and pass through the regulatory review process is an important factor in the cost of development, and so the "drug lag" has a bearing on this cost. There is a clear need to obtain objective and meaningful measures of the rate of new pharmaceutical discovery and development and of the effects of factors such as legislation and regulation on this rate.

A recent study of the economics of the pharmaceutical industry in Britain was performed by the Economic Development Committee for Chemicals. The report of this study pointed out that one of the factors contributing to the attractiveness of the United Kingdom for the development of a pharmaceutical industry was the system for the registration of new medicines. The report also, however, noted that the continuing attractiveness of Britain would depend on, among other factors, "maintenance of the system for the registration of new medicines in its present reasonable and non-bureaucratic form under the new statutory arrangements."[25]

Conclusions

Three general conclusions emerge about the processes of developing and introducing new drugs and about the differences between the British and American approaches.

The first concerns the effects of the "drug lag," based on the evidence currently available. The protection conferred by delaying the introduction of new drugs needs to be weighed against the therapeutic losses thus incurred. From the present evidence, it appears that each country has gained in some ways and lost in others. On balance, however, it is difficult to argue that the United States has escaped an inordinate amount of new drug toxicity by its conservative approach; it has gained little else. On the other hand, it is relatively easy to show that Britain has gained by having effective drugs available sooner. Furthermore, the costs of this policy in terms of damage due to adverse drug reactions have been small compared with the existing levels of damage produced by older drugs. There appear to be no other therapeutic costs of any consequence in Britain. In view of the clear benefits demonstrable from some of the drugs introduced into Britain, it appears that the United States has lost more than it has gained from adopting a more conservative approach than did Britain in the post-thalidomide era.

The second conclusion is a reinforcement of our earlier observations concerning the disproportionate attention given to ascertaining a drug's safety in the earlier phases versus the later phases of its development, and the need to improve postmarketing surveillance. When widespread, catastrophic drug toxicity has occurred, it has only been after a drug has been marketed, and never in the early phases of development. There is a tendency for episodes of this nature to be taken as evidence of laxity in the drug approval process; however, in the present regulatory era when preclinical tests are being used to—and possibly beyond—the limit of their usefulness, it would be more correct to regard widespread toxicity as a failure of postmarketing surveillance than as a failure of premarketing screening.

The appreciation of this fact appears to underlie a major difference in practice between the current drug regulatory systems in the United States and Britain. In the United States, animal and premarketing procedures are generally more demanding than in Britain; implementation of the regulations requires a large number of people; assessment takes a relatively long time. Nationwide postmarketing surveillance is, as we have seen, poorly developed by international standards. In the United Kingdom, the premarketing requirements are less onerous, and new drug applications are processed in quicker time with a considerably smaller staff. Conversely, Britain is compelled to place more reliance on its more sophisticated surveillance system,[26] and this approach appears to have forestalled, with the exceptions noted earlier, widespread toxicity due to the introduction of new drugs. Britain seems to have benefited from this approach.

The third conclusion is that fundamental differences can be discerned in the roles of the regulatory agencies in Britain and the United States, which carry profound implications for the practice of medicine.

In Britain the formal focus of the drug approval process, from the formation of the Committee on Safety of Drugs in 1963 until 1971, was on safety; however, since safety was judged in the context of the intended use of the agent, efficacy was an implicit consideration.[27] Since the implementation in 1971 of the Medicines Act, evidence of efficacy has been explicitly required for approval of a new drug, in addition to the evidence of quality and safety required previously. The current position on efficacy in Britain, as expressed by the Committee on Safety of Medicines (the more powerful successor to the Committee on Safety of Drugs), is that the previous policy will continue:

> The Committee believed that the main purpose of the Act was to provide a safeguard against indiscriminate promotion of dangerously toxic medicines or medicines of inadequate quality, but that it had never been intended that it should be used to deny to the public a large number of products which presented no hazard. . . . It was agreed accordingly to adhere to the policy, originally stated by the Committee on Safety of Drugs in 1965, that "the Committee must consistently consider efficacy in relation to safety." If a medicine not known to be effective were recommended for the treatment of a serious illness for which there was already a satisfactory treatment, this would constitute an

unacceptable risk to the patient. Similarly if a medicine were likely to be quite ineffective in the treatment of any disease for which it was recommended and yet carried the slightest risk to the patient, the Committee would regard it as unsafe for use as recommended.[28]

The important difference between Britain and the United States is that, while efficacy was not ignored in the British regulatory process, the policy has so far been that matters of efficacy—especially relative efficacy—and the control of drug use in the context of specific patients are not the prerogative of a regulatory agency, but are better left to the medical profession aided by the free processes of scientific publication, debate, and education.[29]

CHAPTER X

RECENT DEVELOPMENTS, 1972 TO 1974

In this chapter, we will examine developments in the comparison between Britain and the United States from the beginning of 1972, where the study described in Chapter VII ended, to the end of June 1974. Highlights of the more recent developments through June 1975 are also included. Our purpose here is to determine whether any changes have occurred since 1971 in drug introduction patterns in the U.S. and Britain and in the relationship between them.

Such changes are of interest because, over the past two and a half years, regulatory approaches in both the U.S. and Britain have altered. In Britain, the Medicines Act (1968) became law in 1971, as a result of which the review process for new drugs has become more institutionalized in nature, resembling in some respects that of the U.S. (including, according to some observers, the involvement of a slow-moving bureaucracy). In the U.S., on the other hand, there have been considerable regulatory efforts over the past few years to enlighten the review process for new drugs to bring it into conformity with modern standards of medical practice and scientific thought. One way to determine the relative positions of the regulatory systems in the two countries is to examine their effects on current patterns of new drug introduction. The changes that have occurred in the past three years may also be examined as a challenge-dechallenge trial of the consequences of regulation: if overstringency is a factor in the drug lag, then the 1972-74 adjustments in the two regulatory systems should have somewhat decreased the gap between British and American availability of new drugs.

This chapter is based on a paper contained in *Drug Development and Marketing*, ed. Robert B. Helms (Washington, D. C.: American Enterprise Institute for Public Policy Research, 1975), pp. 165-81.

Table 5

SUMMARY OF NEW DRUG INTRODUCTIONS IN BRITAIN AND
THE UNITED STATES, JANUARY 1972–JUNE 1974

Category	Total Drugs	Mutual		Exclusive	
		U.K. first	U.S. first	U.K.	U.S.
Cardiovascular	7	1	0	5	1
Diuretic	2	1	0	1	0
Respiratory	4	3	0	1	0
Antibacterial and chemotherapeutic	17	2	4	6	5
CNS	15	3	3	6	3
Anesthetic	3	2	0	0	1
Analgesics, etc.	7	0	0	7	0
Gastrointestinal	0	0	0	0	0
Total	55	12	7	26	10

The results are shown in the form of tables using the same headings as in Chapter VII. In addition, we shall use a graphic display to show when, and for how long, drugs were exclusively available in either country. For each therapeutic topic, time is represented horizontally in these graphs, and a horizontal line bisects the field. Those drugs which were exclusively available in the U.K. are plotted above this line and those in the U.S. below. The bar representing each drug extends from the time the drug was marketed until its exclusive availability ceased—usually because the drug was marketed in the other country.

Thus, a preponderance of bars above the line would indicate a British lead, while a preponderance below the line would indicate an American lead. The length of the bar shows how long the disparity persisted. What is important is not so much the number of drugs available, but their identity; this arrangement allows us to see that clearly. One of the main points of these graphs is that a vertical line at any point in time allows us to see at a glance the differences between the range of drugs available in each country at that time.

Specific Drugs

Cardiovascular drugs and antihypertensive therapy (Table 6 and Figure 6). The main drugs used in the treatment of hypertension are, apart from diuretics, those shown in Figure 6. Here we have divided

Table 6
INTRODUCTION OF CARDIOVASCULAR DRUGS

Drug	Date of Introduction		Lead in Years (Months)	
	U.K.	U.S.	U.K.	U.S.
Antihypertensive				
Diazoxide (Hyperstat)	Oct. 1969	Feb. 1973	3(4)	
β-adrenoreceptor antagonist				
Timolol (Blocadren)	June 1974	—		
Sotalol (Beta-Cardone)	June 1974	—		
Antiarrhythmic				
Di-isopyramide (Rythomodan)	Sept. 1972	—		
Bretylium tosylate (Bretylate)	Nov. 1972	—		
Antianginal				
β-blockers, q.v.				
Vasodilators and other				
Naftidrofuryl (Praxilene)	May 1972	—		
Dopamine HCl (Intropin)	—	May 1974		
Hypolipidemic				
Cholestyramine (Questran)	1970	Aug. 1973[a]	3	
Polidexide (Secholex)	May 1974	—		

[a] New indication.

the drugs into a mixed group, largely composed of adrenergic-neurone blocking drugs, and the β-blockers.

In the first group (nondiuretic antihypertensives) there has since 1963 been a steady accumulation of exclusively available drugs in Britain, beginning with bethanidine and debrisoquin and, in 1971, clonidine. These, and the other drugs shown here, were reviewed in the previous chapters.

The β-blockers are one of the major developments in the treatment of both angina and hypertension of the past decade; it is now just ten years since the first papers demonstrating the efficacy of propranolol in hypertension were published. The pattern with β-blockers resembles that of the other antihypertensive agents. There is an accumulation of agents exclusively available in Britain, and none exclusively available in the U.S. Propranolol was first marketed in Britain nine years ago. It was available there exclusively for three years before becoming available in the U.S. When pro-

Figure 6

EXCLUSIVE AVAILABILITY OF CARDIOVASCULAR DRUGS

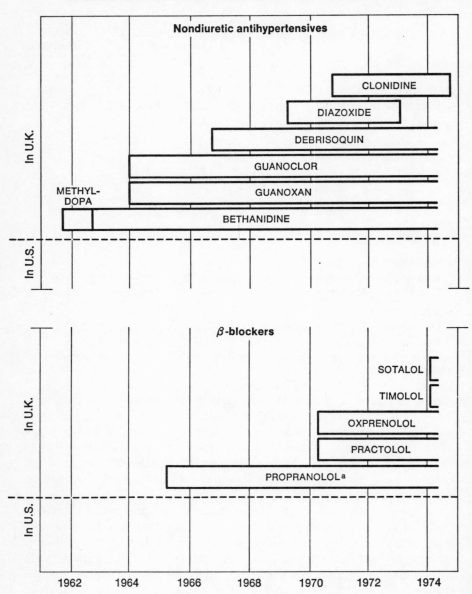

a Not available for angina and hypertension from 1968 to 1973, when it was approved for angina only.

pranolol did become available in the U.S., it was only approved for relatively minor uses; it was not approved for the treatment of angina for a further five years, and it has still not been approved for the therapy of hypertension. This is markedly out of line with expert medical opinion even in the U.S. Then there are other β-blockers that are exclusively available in Britain, some of which offer advantages over propranolol in some patients. Thus, the pattern for the hypertension category is a steady and continuing British lead in the agents available, and the pattern for angina is similar with respect to the β-blockers. The approval of clonidine in the U.S. in 1974 ended one anomaly in this field.

Diuretics (Table 7 and Figure 7). In the group of thiazide and related diuretics there have been no major developments in the last few years, although there are a number of new arrivals which deserve closer comparison with established drugs. The main advances of the past decade are still furosemide and ethacrynic acid, both of which were introduced two years earlier in Britain.

Looking at potassium-sparing diuretics, we find the same pattern: triamterene was marketed first in Britain, and amiloride is still marketed there exclusively.

In view of this, it is hard to understand why slow-release potassium supplements have not been more vigorously sought by industry, government and the profession. The *Medical Letter* continued to criticize the outmoded and dangerous enteric-coated potassium supplements available in the U.S., and the correspondence columns of American journals continued to report disasters due to this dosage form. Meanwhile the number of types of the safer slow-release potassium supplements continues to grow abroad both alone and in combination with diuretics. This hazardous anachronism in the U.S. market persisted for twelve years; the first slow-release potassium supplements were approved for the U.S. market in 1975.

Respiratory drugs (Table 8 and Figure 8). The antiallergic drug cromolyn sodium became available in the U.S. some five and a half years after its introduction in the U.K. This closed one obvious gap, although cromolyn is still available in Britain in dose forms and for indications that have not been approved in the U.S.—for example, for nasal insufflation in the treatment of allergic rhinitis, for which it offers some unique advantages.

An interesting recent development in Britain is the renewed attention being given to corticosteroids by inhalation for the treatment of asthma, as seen in the introduction there of inhaler versions of beclomethasone and betamethasone.

Table 7

INTRODUCTION OF DIURETICS, SLOW-RELEASE K+
SUPPLEMENTS, AND RELATED DRUGS

	Date of Introduction		Lead in Years (Months)	
Drug	U.K.	U.S.	U.K.	U.S.
Diuretic				
Metolazone (Zaroxolyn)	June 1973	Nov. 1973	(5)	
Bumetanide (Burinex)	Sept. 1973	—		
Potassium supplement				
K-Contin	May 1973	—		
Sodium supplement				
Slow sodium	Aug. 1972	—		

This idea is not entirely new. People have for a long time been fascinated by the idea that local application of steroids to the bronchioles would permit local control of allergic bronchospasm by a dose of steroid that was too small to exert much systemic effect, thus eliminating the worst objections to steroid therapy for asthma. Indeed, an inhalable form of dexamethasone has been available for many years on the U.S. market, although it is not at all widely used at present.

What is new is that the concept has now been fairly well vindicated. Relief of bronchospasm occurs with very small doses of steroid. It has been found possible to maintain patients on inhaled, rather than systemic steroids, at very small doses which have much fewer—and, in some cases, no—systemic effects such as adrenal suppression. This is the main advance represented by these newer preparations in use in Britain. Whether the improvements are due to the nature of the steroids, or to refinement of the metered delivery system, or simply to increasing sophistication in the evaluation of these drugs does not seem to have been conclusively established. The main side effect reported so far is candidiasis, and it is not certain yet how serious this side effect will prove in long-term therapy. This development represents a modest advance overall, but one that is of very definite importance to some patients in reducing the systemic side effects of steroids.

The other main area of interest in the respiratory field is that of orally active, longer-acting bronchoselective bronchodilators (see

Figure 7

EXCLUSIVE AVAILABILITY OF DIURETICS AND POTASSIUM SUPPLEMENTS

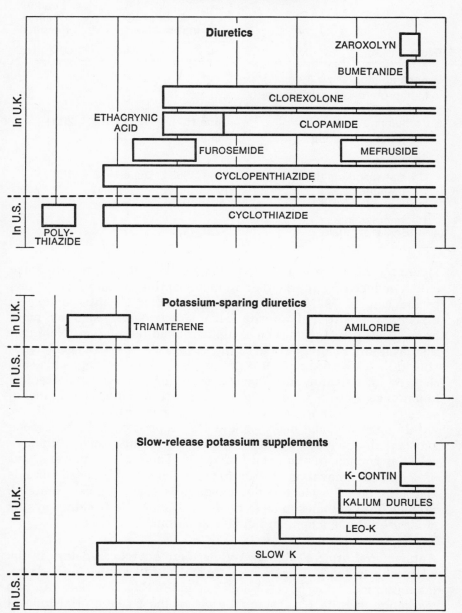

Table 8

INTRODUCTION OF RESPIRATORY DRUGS

Drug	Date of Introduction U.K.	Date of Introduction U.S.	Lead in Years (Months) U.K.	Lead in Years (Months) U.S.
Bronchodilators				
Metaproterenol/orciprenaline (Alupent)	1962	Dec. 1973	11(6)	
Terbutaline (Bricanyl)	June 1971	May 1974	2(11)	
Rimiterol (Pulmadil)	June 1974	—		
Antiallergic				
Cromolyn sodium (Intal, Aarane)	1968	June 1973	5(0)	
Beclomethasone (Becotide inhaler)	Nov. 1972	—		
Betamethasone (Bextasol inhaler)	Sept. 1973	—		

Figure 8). Here the gap between the U.S. and Britain was to some extent reduced by the marketing of metaproterenol (orciprenaline) in the U.S. in 1973, some eleven years after its introduction to Britain, where it had already been largely superseded by more bronchoselective agents such as albuterol and terbutaline. Note that there was still no oral or inhaled highly bronchoselective agent available in the U.S. until mid-1975 (terbutaline). The developments subsequent to metaproterenol have been of less incremental medical importance, but they are all in the direction of increasing bronchoselectivity, with an attendant reduction in acute cardiac side effects.

In summary, the main gaps in the respiratory field have been substantially reduced by the introduction of moderately bronchoselective bronchodilators and cromolyn. There are, however, signs of continued innovation in Britain, particularly with inhaled steroids and more bronchoselective bronchodilators—for example, rimiterol. Bromhexine continues to be exclusively available in Britain, showing modest utility as a sputum liquifier in chronic bronchitis.

Antibacterial drugs (Table 9). While there have been delays in the admission to the U.S. market of several useful antibacterial drugs, the recent marketing of co-trimoxazole in the U.S., five years after its marketing in Britain, substantially clears the backlog of significant drugs in this category which were unavailable in the U.S. Further-

116

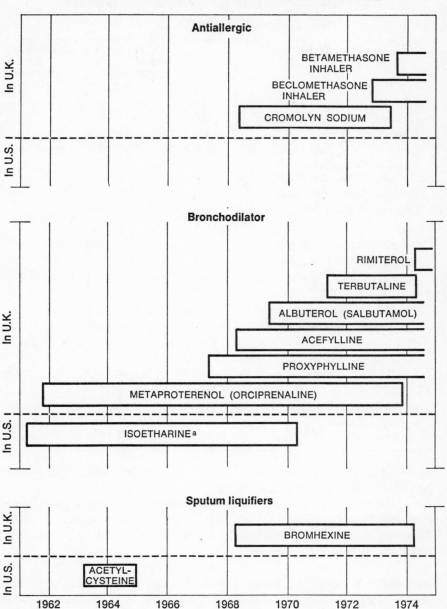

Figure 8

EXCLUSIVE AVAILABILITY OF RESPIRATORY DRUGS

Antiallergic

In U.K.

BETAMETHASONE INHALER

BECLOMETHASONE INHALER

CROMOLYN SODIUM

In U.S.

Bronchodilator

In U.K.

RIMITEROL

TERBUTALINE

ALBUTEROL (SALBUTAMOL)

ACEFYLLINE

PROXYPHYLLINE

METAPROTERENOL (ORCIPRENALINE)

In U.S.

ISOETHARINE a

Sputum liquifiers

In U.K.

BROMHEXINE

In U.S.

ACETYL-CYSTEINE

1962   1964   1966   1968   1970   1972   1974

a Not available as single entity. For details, see W. Wardell, "Introduction of New Therapeutic Drugs in the United States and Great Britain: An International Comparison," *Clinical Pharmacology and Therapeutics*, vol. 14, no. 5 (Sept.-Oct. 1973), p. 781.

Table 9

INTRODUCTION OF ANTIBACTERIAL AND CHEMOTHERAPEUTIC DRUGS

Drug	Date of Introduction U.K.	Date of Introduction U.S.	Lead in Years (Months) U.K.	Lead in Years (Months) U.S.
Penicillins, cephalosporins, etc.				
Amoxicillin (Amoxil)	April 1972	March 1974	2	
Cephradine (Eskacef, Velosef)	Oct. 1972	Aug. 1974	1(10)	
Carbenicillin indanyl sodium (Geocillin Tabs)	—	Nov. 1972		
Cephazolin sodium (Ancef)	June 1974	Oct. 1973		(8)
Cephapirin (Cefadyl)	—	March 1974		
Other				
Co-trimoxazole (Septra, Bactrim)	1968	Sept. 1973	5(3)	
Spectinomycin (Trobocin)	June 1973	Sept. 1971		1(9)
Minocycline (Minocin)	Sept. 1973	1971		2
Antifungal				
Flucytosine (Ancobon)	—	Nov. 1971		
Haloprogin (Halotex Cream)	—	March 1972		
Clotrimazole (Canesten)	Feb. 1973	—		
Miconazole nitrate (Monistat Cream)	June 1974	March 1974		(3)
Antiparasitic				
Nitrimidazine (Nulogyl)	Feb. 1971	—		
Pyrantel pamoate (Antiminth Oral)	—	Jan. 1972		

more, at least two newer antibiotics, spectinomycin and minocycline, have been introduced earlier in the U.S.

In the field of penicillins and cephalosporins, there have been some minor advances in which both countries have shared equally. Thus, in the antibacterial field the gap between the two countries has been virtually eliminated.

Anti-inflammatory analgesics (Table 13 and Figure 9). With the marketing in Britain of six more anti-inflammatory analgesics, there are now eight of these agents exclusively available there.

The medical impact of this is obscure. As far as one can tell, these drugs are all similar in terms of efficacy. The main claim that

Table 10
INTRODUCTION OF ANTICANCER
AND IMMUNOSUPPRESSIVE DRUGS

Drug	Date of Introduction	
	U.K.	U.S.
Thioguanine (Lanvis)	Nov. 1972	—
Bleomycin sulfate (Blenoxane)	—	Aug. 1973
Tamoxifen (Novaldex)	Oct. 1973	—

Table 11
INTRODUCTION OF CENTRALLY ACTING DRUGS

Drug	Date of Introduction		Lead in Years (Months)	
	U.K.	U.S.	U.K.	U.S.
Psychotropic				
Flupenthixol (Depixol)	May 1972	—		
Lorazepam (Ativan)	Feb. 1973	—		
Fluphenazine decanoate (Prolixin Deconoate)	—	April 1973		
Chlorazepate (Tranxene)	Sept. 1973	Sept. 1972	1	
Benperidol (Anquil)	Oct. 1973	—		
Molidone (Moban)	—	March 1974		
Hypnotic				
Flurazepam (Dalmane)	Jan. 1974	Jan. 1971		3
Triclofos (Triclos)	Before 1962	June 1972	10	
CNS stimulant				
Fencamfamin (Reactivan)	June 1971	—		
Muscle relaxant				
Baclofen (Lioresal)	June 1972	—		
Dantrolene (Dantrium)	—	Feb. 1974		
Anorectic				
Fenfluramine (Pondimin)	1964	July 1973	9	
Mazindol (Sanorex)	Jan. 1974	June 1973		(7)
Clortermine (Voranil)	—	June 1973		
Anti-parkinsonism, tremor, etc.				
Benapryzine (Brizin)	Sept. 1973	—		
Carbidopa (Sinemet)	Nov. 1973	May 1975		

Table 12
INTRODUCTION OF ANESTHETIC DRUGS

Drug	Date of Introduction U.K.	Date of Introduction U.S.	Lead in Years (Months) U.K.	Lead in Years (Months) U.S.
General anesthetic				
Trifluoroethyl difluoromethyl ether (Ethrane)	—	Jan. 1973		
Alphaloxone + Alphadolone (Althesin)	July 1972	—		
Local anesthetic				
Bupivacaine (Marcaine)	1968	March 1973	4(9)	
Neuromuscular blocking				
Pancuronium (Pavulon)	1968	Nov. 1972	4(5)	

Table 13
ANALGESIC AND RELATED DRUGS

Drug	Date of Introduction U.K.	Date of Introduction U.S.
Anti-inflammatory analgesic		
Benorylate (Benoral)	Aug. 1971	—
Alclofenac (Prinalgin)	March 1972	—
Naproxen (Naprosyn)	Sept. 1973	—
Ketoprofen (Orudis)	Oct. 1973	—
Fenoprofen (Fenopron)	Feb. 1974	—
Narcotic and narcotic antagonist		
Piritramide (Dipidolor)	June 1972	—
Miscellaneous		
Bufexamac (Feximac)-Topical	Sept. 1973	—

might be made for them is a diminished incidence—or at least a different spectrum—of side effects compared with such classical alternatives as aspirin or phenylbutazone. In the case of some of these drugs, side effects do seem to be less, but the type of proof available is not yet of high standard. There are few rigorous demonstrations of an enhanced therapeutic ratio.

Figure 9

EXCLUSIVE AVAILABILITY OF ANTI-INFLAMMATORY ANALGESICS

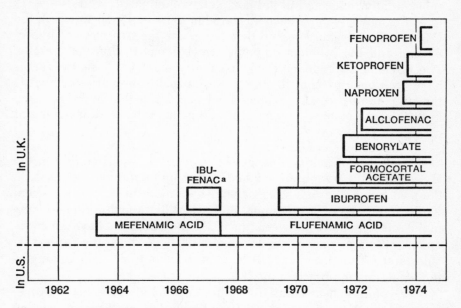

a Ibufenac was withdrawn in Great Britain for toxicity reasons. For details see Wardell, "New Therapeutic Drugs in the United States and Great Britain," p. 785.

One medical effect of this appears to be that there is more use of this class of drug in Britain than in the U.S.; it has been estimated that the per capita utilization rate of anti-inflammatory analgesics in Britain is double that in the U.S. Whether this is, on balance, good or bad is at present unknown.

Gastrointestinal drugs. No new drugs in this category have been marketed in either country since 1971. The British lead in this field remains unchallenged.

Summary and Conclusions

In the study covering the decade through 1971, we found obvious differences between the U.S. and the U.K. in the therapeutic fields represented by cardiovascular, diuretic, respiratory, antibacterial and gastrointestinal drugs. Since then, as our update study shows, this relationship has changed perceptibly in most areas.

In the antibacterial area, the British lead has disappeared, and there is now little difference between the two countries. Some useful new antibiotics have recently been approved earlier in the U.S. than in Britain. In the respiratory field, the previous differences have been substantially reduced, but not completely eliminated, while some interesting new advances have appeared in Britain. Fields in which the U.S. is still noticeably behind Britain include the treatment of hypertension and the problem of potassium balance in diuretic therapy. The obvious discrepancies that currently exist in these two areas have both been present for ten years. A major new development is the large number of anti-inflammatory analgesics that have appeared in Britain, the medical impact of which is unknown and deserving of careful scrutiny.

What can we conclude?

First, it is clear that changes have occurred—particularly in the U.S., where the pattern of available drugs and approved uses has, in the past two and a half years, come to be more in line with current world standards of professional and scientific thought. Some of the major discrepancies between the U.S. and the U.K. have been reduced, although anachronisms remain, particularly in the cardiovascular area. This progress is at least partly due to an enlightening of the regulatory approach in the U.S.

It would be heartening to be able to conclude that this improvement marks the end of a bleak period in American therapeutics and the beginning of a more progressive era. Unfortunately, such a conclusion would be premature, because the FDA has recently come under intense pressure from Congress, from consumer groups, and from factions inside the agency to abandon its medically more realistic attitude.

In March 1974, the FDA was subjected to hearings of the Subcommittee on Intergovernmental Relations, Senate Committee on Government Operations, in which the manner of the FDA's approval process for Depo-Provera and propranolol were criticized. This pressure has continued for these decisions alone, at least through September 1974, in hearings of the Senate Health Subcommittee.

The continuing congressional criticism of the final approval of beta-blockers for angina is destined to become a classic in the history of political pharmacology, with very wide implications for the legislation and regulation of drugs. It is hard to believe that an advisory committee was still debating the approval of this drug for angina when a physician's *failure* to use this drug—for instance as a trial in most patients prior to coronary artery surgery—would be regarded, if not as malpractice, then certainly as substantially suboptimal medical practice.

From the voluminous transcript of these hearings, the criticisms of the FDA in this matter appear to be so out of touch with medical reality that in any other country they could scarcely have seen the light of day in 1964, let alone 1974. For such criticisms to be seriously entertained, there has to be profound ignorance within the medical profession about what is going on in the regulation of drugs.

The FDA in this case has made a long overdue move to bring American regulatory practice into line with the best standards of American medicine, and its action should be strongly supported. The criticism of this action poses a real threat to the very desirable efficacy requirements of the law. If these requirements are implemented in such a manner that they make medical nonsense, than this would obviously impair the credibility of the law in the eyes of physicians and patients to such an extent that the law could be destroyed. For this reason, the recent criticism which undermined the FDA's attempts to adopt a medically sound approach is not only misguided and unwarranted, but a severe disservice to patients. Whatever the outcome, this episode is already a landmark in the annals of food and drug regulation in this country.

Returning to the comparison between Britain and the United States, it is conceivable that the narrowing of the differences between the two countries could be due to a more conservative trend in Britain. The data available do not suggest this yet, but in any case the type of comparison they provide would not be sensitive enough to pick up small changes at an early stage.

Second, the ease with which gross disparities can be detected between countries suggests that some organization ought to be continuously monitoring therapeutic differences between countries. This would be a relatively simple task, but it is one that does not at present seem to be receiving attention. We do not even know much about what is going on in the other English-speaking countries—Canada, Australia, New Zealand, and South Africa—let alone what is happening in foreign-language countries.

Third, these simple and obvious comparisons between countries, although necessary, should be only the beginning of our attempts to chart therapeutic progress and to measure the impact of drugs in absolute therapeutic terms. We need to know how to measure the therapeutic impact, for better or worse, that a new drug has on the community, and—perhaps further in the future—how to assess the potential therapeutic impact of drugs that are prospective candidates for approval.

PART THREE
The Wider Issues

So far in this analysis we have dealt with the evolution of our present system in regulatory, scientific and medical terms and have analyzed the way in which the American solution differs from that of other countries faced with the same problems. With this background, we can proceed to examine fundamental and wider issues.

We shall consider the intent of Congress in the light of the needs of patients and shall attempt to determine whether this intent is, in principle, appropriate for these needs and whether intent and needs are being reconciled in practice. In the light of this, we shall then suggest improvements for our system.

CHAPTER XI

THE INTENT OF CONGRESS
AND THE NEEDS OF PATIENTS

The Intent of Congress

In some ways Congress has been conspicuously successful in the legislation it has created and in the effects of the resulting regulations. The abolition of patent medicines is an outstanding example, as is control over the accuracy of claims made for drugs. Since the 1962 amendments, the advertising of prescription drugs has been effectively controlled to a greater extent here than in most other countries. Untested new medicines are a thing of the past; all the new drugs introduced since 1962 have some proof of efficacy. Totally ineffective medicines are now historical curiosities.

The price of medicines was a special concern of Senator Kefauver. In terms of the benefits attainable with drugs, today's patient is probably getting better value for money than at any time in the past, if only because more drugs actually capable of conferring benefit are continually being developed. Whether this is a result of legislation is a complex question. Peltzman's careful study of the effects of the 1962 amendments suggests that improvement occurred in spite of the regulations, not because of them. According to Peltzman, the new laws have increased the cost of drugs without helping to increase their benefits to any appreciable extent.[1] In any case, legislation has never been aimed at increasing the benefits achievable by drugs. On the contrary, its main thrust has always been to eliminate negative attributes, such as toxicity or ineffectiveness. Positive results, such as encouraging the development of better drugs, have not been specifically sought by legislators or regulators.

In other important respects, Congress has been conspicuously unsuccessful. The requirement that drugs should be tested before marketing has not made them intrinsically safer because, as we shall see, no premarketing tests of safety can substitute for postmarketing surveillance. While premarketing requirements in the United States have become ever more costly and formidable, postmarketing surveillance here is very weak and the United States has had to rely heavily on other countries' surveillance systems. There is also little evidence that the safety of early drug investigation in man has been affected by the 1962 amendments; it is intrinsically a relatively safe process.

Another concern of Congress has been the prevention of monopolies in the pharmaceutical industry. Enforcement of the 1962 amendments has, if anything, entrenched the positions of the biggest firms,[2] since the cost of the drug development process is now such that small companies can rarely develop new products. The duration of patent protection has come under periodic scrutiny. Attempts to reduce monopolistic tendencies by undermining patent protection could endanger the development of new drugs by allowing profits on existing drugs to be reaped by companies that have no intention of doing research. Undermining patent protection not only would reduce incentives to invest in research and development of new drugs, but would also reduce the amount of competition by reducing the flow of new drugs to compete with old ones.

In addition, there are at least two important consequences of its actions that Congress probably did not bargain for. The first of these concerns the development of effective new drugs. By eliminating totally ineffective drugs, the 1962 amendments have ensured that the available drugs are, on average, more effective. But this did not ensure that a greater number of effective drugs would become available. In fact, the opposite happened; the United States came to lag appreciably behind other countries in the introduction of effective new drugs. While it is not possible entirely to untangle legislative, regulatory, industrial and other causative factors in this process, there is no doubt that legislative and regulatory factors, either directly or indirectly, have had a substantial role in the American drug lag, a point made by the FDA itself.[3]

Whether there has been outright suppression of innovation in the United States is a separate and more fundamental question, the answer to which is at present unknown. Techniques for measuring effects in this area are only now being developed. The main requirement the patient has of the drug industry is the development of more effective and safer medicines. Creating conditions inimical to this end was presumably an unintentional step by Congress and the regulatory agency, but it is nevertheless a potentially serious consequence.

The other consequence Congress may not have bargained for when legislating on drug development was the fact that government has come to participate increasingly in the practice of medicine. Attempts to pass judgment on the safety and efficacy of medicines inevitably lead to the assumption of decision-making powers, at a national level by committees of experts, over matters that were formerly regarded as the province of the physician and his patient. Congress initially wished to exert control over the technology of drug assessment; but actions designed to this end inevitably affect the practice of medicine. Denying a physician access to a drug—for example, by preventing it from being marketed—is one example of this; the concept of approved uses is another. While many benefits can result from the participation of government and expert national committees in matters of medical practice, there is potential for harm as well. Such participation is not, therefore, best implemented by adventitious consequences of congressional action aimed at other ends. This is an activity that should be approached with specific aims and appropriate planning.

The Needs of Patients

The patient's primary need is to have a competent, sympathetic and knowledgeable physician who can make best use of the diagnostic, therapeutic, and general resources available in the current state of the art of medicine and who can bring them to bear on the particular needs of that patient. For the purpose of this analysis, we shall confine ourselves to those therapeutic needs of the patient involving drugs. The chief of these needs is a drug, highly effective for his illness, carrying an acceptable degree of risk for the likely benefit to be obtained, and used appropriately by the physician. The patient also has such longer-term but equally clear requirements as the development of new therapies and the finding of safer and more effective ways of using all therapies. It is in every patient's interest, and thus ought to be the intent of Congress, to promote these developments as well. Other requirements are that drugs should be readily available and not disproportionately expensive for the benefits they confer.

Since the patient necessarily has to delegate expert decisions about therapy to his physician, the remainder of this discussion will deal with what a physician needs from drugs in order to treat his patients most effectively. Although we shall continue to confine ourselves to drug-related therapeutics, it should be borne in mind that the issue concerns more than drugs alone; regulatory control is being extended over many other therapeutic and diagnostic procedures and devices. The issues we are dealing with thus affect a large part of medical practice.

Physical properties of drugs. An area where the physician obviously needs third-party assistance is in ensuring that the chemical received by the patient corresponds to the one he prescribed. We have seen the long history of valuable assistance from the pharmacy profession in ensuring accuracy in dispensing and preventing adulteration. In the present century, federal controls have arisen to ensure that the drug dispensed is of defined chemical composition, high purity, and correct weight or potency. The need for federal controls in this area is not seriously questioned by anyone. The achievements of the present legislation and the regulations designed to enforce it, together with the cooperation of industry to achieve these goals, reflect credit on all concerned.

Formulation. In similar fashion, the physician should be able to rely on a third party to guarantee that the dosage form of the drug prescribed is not, like elixir sulfanilamide, intrinsically hazardous, that the dosage form is appropriate for the intended use, and that it will deliver the drug reliably in a known amount and manner. Here again, federal control has proved, for the most part, welcome. However, areas of disagreement arise in setting standards for bioavailability (the amount of active drug made available to the body from a given dosage form and the way in which it is released) and for therapeutic equivalence. Problems arise when a drug's patent expires and other manufacturers seek to market generic forms of it. The biopharmaceutics of a generic manufacturer's product will seldom be identical with those of the original manufacturer's: the generic products may release more or less of their drug, and the resulting blood concentration profile may vary in a number of ways from that of the original. The question is, how close to the original should generics be? Should tolerances be set? Should a generic with superior bioavailability be permitted on the market? While an obvious start would be to impose tolerances—for example, to prevent gross deviations in total bioavailability—one should not be lulled into a false sense of security by this approach. The fundamental problem is that the science of clinical pharmacology has not, so far, been able to elucidate good correlations for most drugs between different blood-level profiles and clinical effect; we seldom know for what precise profiles we should be aiming. It is, therefore, too early to be able to legislate knowledgeably about tolerances for generic products; while tolerances should be an ultimate goal, flexible common sense should apply for the present.

A suggestion has been made that instead of adequate bioavailability, proof of clinical efficacy should be demanded of prospective generic candidates. Even in theory this is not an ideal solution since the statistical power of most clinical studies is so low that, with studies of the size ordinarily feasible, only the grossest differences between active medications can be detected. Furthermore, the vast expense involved in this activity would tend to vitiate the cost savings that are the main object of encouraging generic competition. For example, we recently performed a clinical study of the analgesic efficacy of two forms of methadone.[4] With the size of that study (100 patients) our chance of detecting a real difference of 20 percent in efficacy between the two forms was less than 10 percent. To increase the chance of detection to 95 percent, 4,500 patients would have been required. A study of the latter size would cost over $1 million and need, in our hands, fifty-two years to complete.

Thus, bioavailability and drug equivalence are areas where, while federal controls are desirable in principle, more scientific underpinning is necessary before rigid controls should be imposed.

Efficacy and toxicity. Information about a drug's efficacy and hazards should be freely and readily available to the physician, with expert interpretation where necessary to maximize his ability to choose appropriate therapy for his patients. Furthermore, a drug's potential benefits should be enough to outweigh its hazards in at least some patients.

The work of collecting and communicating to physicians information about a drug's efficacy and hazards must obviously be undertaken on a national scale. Whether direct federal participation is the most effective way of achieving this is arguable. The efforts of the AMA in this field, long before the federal government had any meaningful programs, show that these functions need not necessarily entail legislation or direct government participation.

The methods currently employed by government to compile and disseminate such information also need evaluation. Most government activity centers on the drug's labelling (the package insert). Although the medical usefulness of this has improved markedly in the past year, as seen in the inserts describing cromolyn sodium and co-trimoxazole, it is still primarily a document designed to serve a legal purpose. For example, the exhaustive listing of even rare toxic effects with no relative incidence figures is clinically misleading. The contrast between package inserts and the more realistic descriptions in the AMA's *Drug Evaluations* and in independent publications from many countries illustrates the fundamental difference between legal or quasi-legal documents and primarily medical communications.

How to balance a drug's benefits against its hazards is the fundamental issue. Ultimately these risk-benefit decisions must be made by individual physicians treating individual patients. Unless national committees can anticipate all possible clinical situations that may arise, any action they take to exclude or delay the access of a potentially useful drug to the market will tie the hands of some physicians and risk denying benefits to at least a few patients.

A fundamental distinction exists between the technology of drug assessment and the practice of medicine, despite important areas of overlap. The former aims to elucidate the properties of the drugs and necessarily involves populations of patients, whereas the latter deals with the management of individual patients. The individual nature of practice should not absolve physicians of the need to consider scientific data about the drugs they use; conversely, society's justifiable urge to codify the technological aspects of drug assessment and to establish scientific facts about the efficacy of drugs should not eclipse the fact that it is ultimately individual patients who are to be treated. Perhaps the dichotomy is merely due to technical inadequacies, which will disappear as the science of clinical pharmacology improves. Until then, however, the significance of this distinction should not be underestimated; it is a fundamental cause of the dilemma with which this volume is concerned.

Is the Intent of Congress Compatible with the Needs of Patients?

No one would deny that the provisions of the 1938 law governing tests of safety prior to marketing and the provisions of the 1962 amendments governing investigational plans, proof of efficacy, and control over advertising are in principle and intent compatible with the need of the patient to obtain maximally effective and safe therapy. But are patients' needs being met in practice?

What is good for the majority is not always best for each person; further, problems have arisen in the way in which the law has come to be implemented by regulations. One problem which we shall examine is the difficulty, in the present state of the art of clinical pharmacology, in determining what is meant by the terms *safety* and *efficacy*. Even if such scientific decisions could be made easily, a fundamental problem remains in the sometimes irreconcilable conflict between the needs of a particular individual and those of the whole society. What, for example, should be done about drugs that are essential to a few people but have a high incidence of adverse reactions? No perfect policy can be devised in this situation.

There is evidence, however, that the policies adopted so far have not produced optimal results, nor even—in some instances—the results intended. The key issue is how to determine the point where accommodations are to be made between safety and efficacy in the approval of drugs for the market. Another major problem is how to obtain the greatest benefit and safety with existing drugs while preserving the incentives and capacity for the pharmaceutical industry to create better ones. There are many variants of this problem. What should be done about the lack of incentive for industry to develop those new drugs which may be major breakthroughs but have only a very small market? What should be done with older drugs: should money and effort be spent on applying to them the same standards of efficacy as totally new drugs must meet? What would be the benefit to society of requiring massive expenditure on this pedestrian and questionably desirable activity, since it would divert funds from discovering and evaluating new and possibly more useful drugs? Similar considerations apply to combination drugs and over-the-counter preparations.

CHAPTER XII

THE RUBRICS REEXAMINED

In the debate over how new therapeutic drugs should be developed and introduced, certain guidelines are accepted by most parties without question. The purpose of this chapter is to examine three such rubrics: (1) "Therapeutic drugs should be proven to be safe and effective for their intended uses before being permitted on the market." (2) "Committees of experts are better able to judge the safety, efficacy and appropriate usage of drugs than are individual physicians." (3) "Access of a drug to the market is the most appropriate point at which to control drug utilization."

Should Therapeutic Drugs Be Required to Be Proven Safe and Effective for Their Intended Uses before Being Permitted on the Market?

This is a thoroughly laudable goal, but it is at present unattainable. This rubric depends on three prior assumptions.

The assumption that "the terms safety and efficacy have been adequately defined." The fact is that safety and efficacy have never been defined in operational terms suitable for the science of drug evaluation. Even if they had been so defined, we would still lack objective criteria for deciding how much is enough of either quality.

Feinstein has pointed out our current inadequacies, which include the tendency to think in terms of statistical rather than clinical significance, our inability to evaluate multiple drug effects and in particular to weigh diverse beneficial effects against equally diverse toxic effects, our disregard of the total therapeutic situation in our concern for obtaining scientifically respectable data on drug efficacy with resultant information that is dehumanized and clinically often of doubtful value, and our currently inadequate attention to such matters as comorbidity, prognostic stratification, and the problem of extrapolating from the results of clinical trials to the population at large.[1]

Until the science of drug evaluation has been developed to the point where it is fully relevant clinically, it is premature to adopt a rigidly legalistic approach to matters of drug efficacy and safety. Indeed, the wording of the present law is relatively broad in its specification; it is the interpretation that tends to become too rigid.

There has been disagreement with this argument on the grounds that it represents a threat to the law's efficacy requirement. This, it is asserted, will drag us back to the dark ages of medical therapy, encouraging physicians to tinker recklessly with the modern pharmaceutical equivalents of leeches, bloodletting and purging. We are not so pessimistic, because the argument is not against the law itself, which is very broad in its wording, but against unrealistically rigid interpretation of the law.

A revealing illustration of our present inability to handle scientifically meaningful concepts of drug safety and efficacy by means of legally watertight definitions emerged during congressional subcommittee hearings, already referred to, on the manner in which certain drugs—notably propranolol—had been approved for use in 1973.

Most of the debate between the pharmaceutical industry and the Food and Drug Administration stems from disagreement as to what constitutes evidence of safety and efficacy, whether the available data satisfy the present perceived requirements, whether a particular degree of safety or efficacy is sufficient for the intended use, and what uses should be deemed appropriate. We are deluding ourselves by suggesting that safety and efficacy are adequately or even clearly defined concepts in the present state of the art of clinical pharmacology.

The answer is to ensure that the law and regulations do not overstep the current capabilities of the science, and at the same time to work to improve the ability of the underlying science to contribute to medically meaningful decisions on drugs. If all parties take this approach with the patient's welfare always in mind, it would seem to represent progress rather than a return to the dark ages.

The foregoing considerations apply to the relatively straightforward question of assessing safety and efficacy in order for a drug to be allowed on the market. After drugs have been marketed, the problem of measuring safety and efficacy is much more difficult. While there are some crude methods for measuring the overall hazards of drugs under conditions of actual use, methods for measuring the overall benefits that drugs produce under the same conditions hardly exist. For the most part we have neither the techniques nor the data for making the risk-benefit decisions that need to be made about drugs under conditions of actual use.

The assumption that "appropriate uses can be clearly distinguished from inappropriate uses by a central authority." One must distinguish between the need for regulatory agencies to determine appropriate use for the population as a whole and the need for individual physicians to determine appropriate use in particular patients. Frequently, due to the trial-and-error nature of much therapeutics in the current state of the art, the appropriateness of a particular drug use for a given patient can only be known empirically. "Appropriate use" as a concept is therefore not as strong in a community context as it is in an individual one. Individual physicians are better placed to determine appropriate use than are national committees.

Two examples of this are the restricted (or "approved") uses of propranolol and carbamazepine in the United States. Although both drugs are marketed in the U.S., they were not originally approved here for use in some of their major indications in the rest of the world: hypertension and, until September 1973, angina in the case of propranolol, and, until August 1974, epilepsy in the case of carbamazepine. There is no doubt about the efficacy of either compound when used in appropriate patients;[2] in any case, the clinical management involves direct scrutiny of efficacy in each patient. There is also no doubt that these drugs can be toxic. Propranolol's toxicity is dose-dependent, predictable and reversible; carbamazepine's is capricious.

The important point is that the decision to use either agent is, like any therapeutic decision in medicine, an intensely individual one that must weigh the risks and benefits for a particular patient. It is unlikely that the approval of some uses and disapproval of others on a community-wide basis will be in the best interests of all patients. Wide experience in other countries,[3] and the reaction of expert physicians and the American Medical Association[4] in the United States, speaks to the contrary.

The assumption that "safety, efficacy, and appropriateness of use can be determined prior to the point of marketing." Leaving aside for the moment the difficulty of establishing the safety, efficacy, and appropriate use of drugs, we now consider whether any such determinations can be made prior to the point of marketing. Here preclinical (animal) and clinical tests need to be dealt with separately.

Do the results of preclinical tests of a drug in animals have predictive value for determining safety and efficacy of that drug in man? While substantial faith is placed in it, the predictive value of animal tests has seldom been critically examined. One of the very few empirical studies of this point to date is that of Litchfield. Surveying six drugs of dissimilar chemical structure that had been extensively evaluated in the rat, dog, and man, Litchfield found that more than half the toxic effects in man had been entirely missed by the animal screens, while at least a fifth of the positive predictions of toxicity were incorrect. At least with the methods in use at that time, animal tests in both rodent and non-rodent species could not be relied upon to predict a drug's toxicity in man.[5] Other examples exist to reinforce this point.[6]

Animal testing requirements should not exceed those necessary to protect the humans in the next study contemplated. A corollary of this is that we should know what degree of protection we are actually achieving with animal tests. We have already seen that predictive tests based on animals do not remove all risk for man. Some of the data needed needed to illuminate this problem exist, but they are in the files of industry and the regulatory agencies, where they have not hitherto been available. We still need to know precisely what risks are incurred by those humans who take a new compound in its early clinical stages and to what extent the use of prior animal tests alters those risks. This will include determining at what stage of clinical testing, early or late, the most serious human toxicity occurs.

Against this we need to weigh how the criteria used for performing and interpreting animal tests affect the likelihood of discarding useful compounds. The lethal effect of penicillin on two animal species was only discovered some years after its introduction to human medicine. Sir Alexander Fleming once remarked that the success of the penicillin project depended on the fact that, since he was not a pharmacologist, he had not tested the drug in animals at all and that, knowing in retrospect its animal toxicity, he would never have had the courage to try it on man![7] If even one new drug of the stature of penicillin or digitalis has been unjustifiably banished to a company's back shelf because of excessively stringent animal requirements, that event will have harmed more people than have been affected by all the toxicity that has occurred in the history of modern drug development. It is entirely conceivable that the losses from excessively conservative interpretation of animal toxicity tests are more harmful than the toxicity that would be experienced if drugs were tested in man, with appropriate safeguards, at an earlier stage.

Are there adequate safeguards at either industrial or regulatory levels in the existing drug development process to prevent potentially valuable drugs from being discarded at the preclinical stage? There appear to be none; the present system seems designed to pave the way for errors of this type. We do not know how many valuable compounds have been lost to man in this way, but an instructive example is the uniquely active antischistosomal compound SQ18,506.[8] If really exhaustive animal testing is to be required, the most efficient place for it is after a compound has been shown, by brief early human studies, to have some promise in man. Our approach to preclinical requirements should take this into account in a fashion consistent with the protection of the human subjects.

Does exhaustive premarketing evaluation of drugs in man protect the public from subsequent widespread hazard? There is surprising faith in the belief that important side effects in man can reliably be detected at an early stage and that sufficiently intensive study of a drug in its premarketing phase in some way confers protection after the drug is marketed. Neither of these views is correct.

In the first place, the number of patients that can feasibly be studied intensively in the investigational stages of a drug's history are limited. Hence the only side effects that can be detected at all in the premarketing stage are those that occur very frequently. Premarketing studies of any realistic size have very little chance of detecting rare but important side effects. For example, to have a 95 percent chance of detecting a side effect with a frequency of one in one hundred—and catastrophic side effects are typically several orders of magnitude less frequent than this—300 patients would be necessary.[9] Recent discussion of the requirements for evaluation of combination antibiotic ophthalmological preparations has indicated that upwards of 15,000 patients would be required to detect the anticipated differences in eye infection rates.[10] Bone marrow toxicity of the chloramphenicol or phenylbutazone type, with a frequency of one in 20,000 or smaller, would simply not be detectable with any feasible premarketing testing.

A similar argument applies to efficacy, as exemplified by our own study, previously referred to, on the statistical power of analgesic evaluation.

Since widespread, catastrophic, drug toxicity can be recognized only after the drug has been marketed, and since, as we have previously shown, new drugs contribute only a small part of the overall burden of drug toxicity, preventive measures must be aimed at both new and old drugs *in the circumstances of their actual use. Premarketing observations, no matter how intense, can never be an adequate substitute.*

Current procedures of drug development in the United States seem to be based on the exact opposite of this logic. Preclinical and premarketing testing is becoming increasingly more demanding, while postmarketing surveillance is essentially neglected. The United States reporting rate is among the lowest of all twelve countries reporting to the WHO International Drug Monitoring Program,[11] and meaningful feedback from the monitoring system in the United States to the physicians who are in a position to contribute was nonexistent until 1974. A similarly gloomy assessment of the FDA's current handling of adverse reaction reporting was made by the U.S. General Accounting Office (GAO) in 1974.[12]

Our conclusion is that satisfactory objective criteria of safety and efficacy do not yet exist, and in any case they cannot be exhaustively or meaningfully defined prior to the point of marketing.

Are Committees of Experts Better Able to Judge the Safety, Efficacy, and Appropriate Usage of Drugs than Are Individual Physicians?

This rubric illustrates the difference in the approach of a regulatory agency, which seeks to optimize the use of therapeutic tools for the community as a whole, and of the individual physician, who seeks to use those tools in a way best for individual patients. There will always be some conflict here, because in the real world drugs will be used imperfectly by some physicians. It is probable that the more therapeutic decisions are assumed by expert committees, the more will minorities of patients suffer. However, no study has ever been made to determine how much collective decision making in this area benefits the majority, and whether its harm to minorities is small enough to be ignored. If, for example, a use is not approved, directions for that nonapproved use and appropriate dosage forms will not be available even to specialist physicians who want to use the drug for such purposes in patients with unusual problems. Expert decisions, furthermore, are seldom unanimous.

The consequences of the trend towards collective decision making deserve to be explored further. It will always result in timorous policies; under public scrutiny, regulatory bodies tend to make excessive allowance for worst-case possibilities. Such policies have helped to create the American drug lag and the associated restrictions on uses for those drugs that are released.

Is Access of a Drug to the Market the Most Crucial and Appropriate Point at which to Exert Control over Drugs?

The real object of controls over the marketing of therapeutic drugs lies, paradoxically, not in the control of marketing per se, but in control of the way in which drugs are used therapeutically. It has never been proved—and seems unlikely on the face of it—that control over marketing is the best way to control drug utilization.

All drugs have hazards if they are used inappropriately; control over marketing tends to exclude even those effective though hazardous drugs which benefit some patients if used appropriately. The key issue should not be how to control the marketing of a useful but toxic drug, but how to ensure that it is used appropriately.

If controls over the admission of drugs to the market are imperfect, one ought to examine alternative methods. Examples exist in which utilization controls have proved to be more precise and yet more flexible than controls over the access of a drug to the market. In New Zealand, for example, a national health service which includes government payment for pharmaceuticals has existed for thirty-six years. For most of this time there was no control over the access of drugs to the market. Instead, powerful controls have always been exerted at an alternate point, namely the manner in which drugs are utilized in general practice.[13] These controls stem from the conditions required for the patient to obtain drugs free of charge under the government's Pharmaceutical Benefits Scheme. The controls include restriction of certain drugs to supply by hospital pharmacies, to prescription by specialists, and to use in approved indications, and limitations on the duration of supply on a single prescription. None of these restrictions apply in hospitals or to the patient who is prepared to pay for the drug himself; all can be waived on application by the doctor to the Department of Health. The effectiveness of these measures has been demonstrated. For example, New Zealand was almost completely spared the thalidomide tragedy because of utilization controls at a time when no marketing controls existed. Although available for two years, the drug had not been admitted to the Drug Tariff and so was not paid for by the Health Service. Controls over utilization probably protect the New Zealand patient considerably more than controls over marketing protect the American patient, since utilization controls extend to all hazardous drugs, new or old (for example, chloramphenicol). A somewhat similar, but more recent, system of utilization controls based on government reimbursement exists in Australia.

We are not suggesting that systems of this type would necessarily be better for the American patient; this example is used solely to point out that in concentrating on control over marketing, Congress and the public may have missed the point.

Thus, it is by no means obvious that access to the market is the most appropriate place to exert control over drugs, nor that strict control over marketing can provide for the best utilization; neither is it necessarily clear that a regulatory agency is the most appropriate tool to exert such control.

We must conclude that some of the rubrics of our present system are logically precarious, while others are impractical. Since there apparently is no unequivocally correct way to proceed, alternative approaches to the control of drug development ought to be explored.

CHAPTER XIII

SUGGESTIONS FOR IMPROVEMENT

In the previous chapter, we showed that the apparently reasonable rubrics which underlie our current attitudes towards drug development have substantial logical and practical defects. Here we shall explore some areas in which improvements are possible, bearing in mind that society's main needs are for improved drugs to be developed and for all drugs to be used in the best manner possible. Any new legislation should focus on these goals.

Stimulate Discovery and Development

Innovation. In order to stimulate drug innovation, one must be able to measure the output of the innovative process and understand the factors responsible for it so that these can be made to produce maximum social benefit.

With a few exceptions such as the U.S. National Cancer Institute (NCI), the only source of therapeutic drug discovery and development in the U.S. is the pharmaceutical industry. This creativity is the industry's most valuable and unique contribution to society. Society should recognize this fact and should seek to foster innovative research.

Since we know relatively little about the innovative process, we need independent research into its steps and elements. The international comparisons described in this volume are only a start; much more is needed.

We need to understand the basic process of innovation itself—as measured, for example, by the rate of synthesis of new chemical structures, the rate of investigation of these in animals and man, and the flow of significant new drugs to the market. The earlier steps in this process have received practically no attention, and data are generally unobtainable for reasons of confidentiality. In addition, we need to know about the mechanisms of the decision-making process within firms and the role that internal and external factors play in influencing such decisions.

We particularly need to examine the effect of legislative and regulatory policies on drug discovery and development. The idea of requiring research impact statements,[1] analogous to environmental impact statements, is an attractive one. Legislators have tended to overlook the need for better drugs in their justifiable concern to protect the public against drug-induced harm. It is sobering to note that the Food, Drug and Cosmetic Act [2] devotes no specific attention to our need to improve upon the drugs we already have.

It should be clearly recognized that existing drugs are inadequate to deal with most of the diseases we face. The object of legislation in this area should be to protect the patient against all diseases, not just iatrogenic ones. The public interest would be well served by policies designed to stimulate the development and introduction of better medicines. This has already been recommended by the President's Science Advisory Committee.[3] It would be a historic and entirely feasible step if government agencies, including the FDA, were given formal mandates to do this.

Such reasoning ultimately leads to the idea that government should support or participate in drug research and development, in particular for therapy that is not commercially attractive.[4] Government support was favorably considered in a report by a working party of the Chemicals Economic Development Committee of the British National Economic Development Council, which is the national forum for economic consultation between government, management and unions.[5]

There are already precedents for such U.S. pharmaceutical research and development in the U.S. Army's antimalarial drug program and the National Cancer Institute's antitumor drug program.

Dr. Gordon Zubrod, while director of the Division of Cancer Treatment at the NCI, testified that one of the main differences between government-supported and industry-supported research is that the NCI's mission

> tends to be much broader than that of private industry. The pharmaceutical house must limit drug development to those areas that are of direct interest to the company, while the focus of the NCI program is upon the patient. We are charged with following every lead for active drugs, even though these may be of benefit to relatively small numbers

144

of patients, and we do this with leads developing not only in the United States, but across the whole world. Therefore a number of anti-tumor drugs have been developed in which industry would not have been interested.[6]

It should be noted that even the NCI, with hundreds of drugs at the IND stage, has never brought a drug to market nor even filed an NDA.

After carrying out much of the clinical workup of certain drugs, the NCI offers them for licensing to the pharmaceutical industry. Even then, despite such assistance, the commercial promise of a drug is often not attractive enough to tempt prospective manufacturers.[7] This should warn us that drug research and development that is not commercially attractive may ultimately become unattractive to government-sponsored research institutions as well.

Intellectual incentives for innovation should not be ignored. Clinical drug research occupies an enormous amount of medical talent in industry and in the academic and professional communities. A vast amount of this work is of necessity pedestrian, with only a relatively small amount involving innovative and intellectually pioneering activities. If the regulatory thrust is too far in the direction of satisfying routine requirements, we will risk wasting precious innovators on such work or even diverting them from the field altogether. It has been stated, for example, that the industry's need to defend older drugs whose marketability is threatened by the drug efficacy review has diverted resources from drug innovation. Regulatory policy should recognize the fact that innovative intellects are to be encouraged rather than suppressed, and that the field of drug development needs to be seen as a challenging and attractive career for academic and other physicians.

Realistic premarketing requirements. Since we have seen that the available methodology is not ideal either for discovering new drugs or for safeguarding patients, we consider here how both processes may be improved.

Because of the peculiar social, ethical, and political problems involved in drug development, there is a tendency to give more weight to a drug's potential hazards than to its potential benefits.

There are several instructive examples of drugs that reached the market before the full extent of their human or animal toxicity was appreciated.[8] It is highly likely, for example, that if all the toxic properties in animals of digitalis, aspirin and fluroxene were appreciated and these drugs appeared today as potential new drug candidates, they would be abandoned; we have already referred to Fleming's own account of the development of penicillin. There are also examples in which the appearance of some toxicity during the development process of an undeniably effective new drug has been allowed to overshadow the benefits of that drug, causing unnecessary delay or abandonment. Examples of this are gentamicin [9] and the antischistosomal drug SQ18,506; there are many other examples seen in our study of the drug lag.

Since the desired goal is to have human investigation begin as early as is consistent with safety, we now examine the risks of drug evaluation in man and the safeguards needed.

These risks depend in part upon what stage has been reached in the drug's history. At the earliest stages, when the drug is being tested for tolerance, little risk is permissible because the subjects have nothing to gain from the procedure; at the later stages, when efficacy has already been demonstrated, more risk is tolerable as the potential benefits to the patient mount. Eventually, investigational use will merge into therapeutic use as more about the drug becomes known. Conversely, all drugs, even old ones, should be regarded as investigational, since we should never be satisfied with the available knowledge.

Thus it is the earliest studies in man that give rise to the most ethical problems. How hazardous is it, then, to receive a new drug?

Although the earliest studies of a drug in man are commonly thought to be the most dangerous, the subjects in these studies are the most carefully monitored, and serious toxicity in fact seldom occurs at this stage. There is some evidence to suggest that the earliest studies are the safest, but we cannot tell whether this safety has been achieved because of animal screening or in spite of it. Carr summarized experience, predominantly with Phase I studies, at one prison testing unit in Michigan where nearly 14,000 volunteers participated in more than 300 studies during a seven-year period without any occurrence of serious toxicity.[10] A recent FDA survey [11] confirms the safety of early drug investigation since the 1962 amendments. Obviously, more hard data on this topic, particularly concerning the nature and reversibility of reactions that do occur and the documentation of long-term sequelae, are needed. There is no doubt, however, that when widespread toxicity occurs, it is not in the early stages of a drug's development, since its use is at that point restricted to small numbers of people and is extremely closely supervised. Widespread toxicity can only occur after a drug has been approved for marketing, when it comes to be used over a long period and in relatively unsupervised fashion by large numbers of patients. A corollary of this is that surveillance should be intensified at all levels of drug investigation and use, but particularly in the post-marketing phase.

Improve Drug Utilization

If all drugs were used perfectly, few constraints on the process of drug development, and none on utilization, would be necessary. The improvement of drug utilization is thus of special importance. Here we shall consider methods of improvement at both the premarketing and the postmarketing stages.

Effective Surveillance. Early human trials, together with closer and more scientific surveillance and follow-up of drugs in man, are preferable to excessive reliance on animal tests; but surveillance must extend far beyond the point of marketing. Just as preclinical toxicity testing can never guarantee a drug's safety in man, neither can the small numbers of closely monitored patients who participate in premarketing trials guarantee its safety in the population at large. For this reason, the actions of a regulatory agency should hinge to a significant degree on the quality of postmarketing surveillance. If this is poor or nonexistent, then the decision to approve a new drug is a grave and essentially irreversible one and should be delayed as long as possible. If, on the other hand, postmarketing surveillance is rigorous enough to detect even rare and mild toxicity in man at an early stage, then drugs can be approved much more rapidly, with confidence that prompt action on information from the surveillance system will forestall any great harm to the community even if the drug does turn out to have unsuspected hazards. There is abundant evidence, including the GAO report already referred to, that postmarketing surveillance has been inadequate in the U.S.

An obvious improvement, now receiving attention in the United States, is to market a drug initially in a gradual, monitored fashion instead of the customary all-or-none, unmonitored manner.[12] If the initial release of new drugs were restricted to individuals or institutions with special facilities to monitor them, drugs could be released at a considerably earlier stage than at present. A procedure of this type has been incorporated into some of the systems of utilization controls to be described later.

A few drugs have been released, or release has been proposed, under monitored or restricted conditions in the U.S.—for example, levodopa, methadone for maintenance programs, Depo-Provera, and Ethrane. The success of such schemes will, however, require a change of attitude and increased sympathy from the pharmaceutical industry and from the medical and pharmacy professions, because it sets up restrictions on who can use new drugs. Restrictions on methadone distribution, for example, were overthrown on legal grounds after a suit was filed by pharmacists.

One aspect of postmarketing surveillance is to monitor the experience of other countries. This has much to recommend it, particularly for drugs released in countries with good surveillance systems, although excessively conservative policies would tend to result, since these systems currently measure only hazards and not benefits.

The resources available to develop and regulate new drugs are not unlimited. Excessive reliance on animal screening and premarketing clinical trials is not the best way to use these resources. Society would benefit more from directing a greater proportion of effort toward responsive clinical drug surveillance than from raising the preclinical and premarketing hurdles still higher.

Therapeutic Uses of Unmarketed Drugs

We propose the creation of a distinction between the therapeutic and the investigational use of yet unmarketed drugs. In addition, we advocate earlier but restricted release of certain drugs for therapeutic purposes.

The object of investigation of a new drug under the IND procedure is to obtain evidence of the drug's properties in order to satisfy the law. The purpose of the IND procedure is not to treat disease or to help specific patients; indeed, at present it actually hinders patients' access even to therapies that are known to be beneficial to them.

Important new drugs must go through an IND-NDA process lasting several years before being marketed in the U.S.; they have often been available abroad for some years before investigation even began in the U.S. Any drug that benefits patients after marketing in the U.S. would have been equally helpful to those same patients *before* its marketing date. The act of NDA approval does not confer activity on a hitherto inactive drug; it simply recognizes activity that the drug has always possessed. Therefore, there will always be drugs that are as yet unmarketed in the U.S. but that would nevertheless benefit some patients here.

Individual patients who genuinely need such a drug have no guaranteed access to it in this country. They are entirely dependent on the sponsoring company, whose primary aim must be to satisfy the NDA requirements. If no company or other sponsor has yet filed an IND application, or if a sponsoring company is unwilling to allow the drug to be used outside its own program, then the patient's problem is much more difficult. Short of the patient or his physician filing a private IND application, which can require complete chemical and animal data, there is no practical way for a patient to obtain that drug legally in the U.S. at all. In any case, possession of a private IND exemption does nothing toward obtaining the drug from an unwilling company.

This is not an optimal state of affairs. Indeed, it is contrary to the Declaration of Helsinki adopted by the eighteenth World Medical Assembly in 1964 which, under the heading "Clinical Research Combined with Professional Care," states: "1. In the treatment of the sick person, the doctor must be free to use a new therapeutic measure if, in his judgement it offers hope of saving life, re-establishing health, or alleviating suffering."

There is an obvious need to ensure that the procedures for governing the investigational use of new drugs in the U.S. do not hinder the therapeutic use of those drugs for patients who really need them. Clearly, safeguards have to be set up so that the use of a drug for therapeutic purposes does not preclude the acquisition of the scientifically acceptable information necessary for the NDA. It would therefore be desirable to keep therapeutic use within the framework of the IND process. This would need considerable modification of our approach to the IND procedure, including the question of whether a drug's sponsor should have absolute control over how it is to be used in this phase. In the proper scientific framework, the therapeutic use of investigational drugs could do much to improve the utilization of very new drugs. It would, furthermore, remove some of the conflict between the practicing physician, who wishes to prescribe the best therapy for individual patients, and the regulatory agency, which wishes to deal with drugs on a community-wide basis.

An intriguing and probably controversial point regarding the standard of evidence needed for NDA approval arises from this line of argument. In many clinical situations, it is quite easy to establish the efficacy of a therapy in a specific patient; this is, indeed, a necessary and routine part of good therapeutic practice. If this empirical procedure were refined into a crossover experiment with appropriate controls, one could establish unequivocally whether the drug is active in that patient. By such a rigorous demonstration in one patient, the drug has indeed been shown to have efficacy. Such a situation would arise, for example, if agents like Vitamin B_{12}, insulin, or thyroid hormone were being studied for the first time in appropriate patients. Evidence of this type would technically satisfy the efficacy requirements of the law for "well controlled investigations, including clinical investigations."

Examples do exist of the distinction between therapeutic and investigational uses of new drugs. In the U.S., the National Cancer Institute has used the IND procedure extensively for purely therapeutic drug use. Zubrod testified as follows:

> In regard to anti-tumor drugs, I would call attention to one major problem, namely, the long time lag that exists between the point at which the professionals become convinced by the data generated under an IND, that a new drug is truly helpful to cancer patients, and the approval of the NDA. [A number of reasons for this are given.] . . .
>
> The impact of this lag has not been of serious import in the cancer field because *our widespread research network allows us to supply drugs to a fairly large number of patients. . . .*
>
> Until an NDA is granted, the NCI must be responsible for seeing that every patient who needs a drug will get it. If we are the sole distributors of a drug, it is unjustifiable to withhold the drug from patients who need it[13] [emphasis supplied].

However, in reference to the drug adriamycin, "one of the most active anti-tumor drugs under present study [and one for which U.S. IND] studies confirm British experience," Zubrod notes that it "is being used throughout our research network, but the drug reaches *only a small fraction of those patients who could benefit from it*"[14] [emphasis supplied]. As shown earlier, adriamycin, already marketed in Britain at the time of Zubrod's remarks, was finally approved in the U.S. in 1974, after being approved in thirty-one other countries previously.

The NCI is a unique case in the U.S.: a large government program, implemented at 200 institutions throughout the country, is being used to bypass the obstacles set up by the law's IND procedures in order to help individual patients obtain promptly the fruits of modern research; however, by its director's own testimony, even these substantial efforts are inadequate. Comparable procedures do not even exist for making investigational drugs therapeutically available to patients in other disease areas.

Zubrod's suggestions for improvement include earlier limited approval (monitored release), simplification of the NDA process for drugs whose efficacy is already well documented—for example, abroad—and more positive action on approving new uses for already marketed drugs.

Distinction between investigational and therapeutic use of new drugs is provided for in the British Medicines Act of 1968, which excludes from its scope the treatment of individual patients by physicians. Section 9 of the act, referring to its general provisions and exemptions, states that "the restrictions . . . do not apply to anything done by a doctor or dentist which (a) relates to a medicinal product . . . [prepared or imported] . . . for administration to a particular patient of his. . . ." [15]

Section 31 of the act requires licensing and certification for the investigational use of drugs, but Paragraph 5 of that section exempts from this requirement, in language similar to Section 9, a physician acting on his own behalf to administer any drug to his own patients.

This recognition of a distinction between therapeutic and investigational drug use, which is not widely appreciated, represents a fundamental difference between the American and British approaches to the regulation of new drugs. A distinction similar to the British one seems also to be recognized in the Swedish system of drug regulation.

Methods of influencing utilization. In the United States, two main methods are used to control drug utilization. One is control over the access of drugs to the market: new drugs can be denied access and old drugs can be removed from the market if they are deemed to be unsafe or ineffective. The other type of control is over the way marketed drugs are used, exerted mainly through the drugs' labeling.

For the control of foodstuffs—from which this approach is derived—labeling is admirable. Control of drug labeling has certain attractive features, such as supervision of content and promotion. However, labeling has begun to be used more broadly than initially envisaged, as in the control of physicians' behavior in specific therapeutic situations. Here, labeling approaches the character of a code of approved practice from which deviations can be measured.

The sanctions underlying this control are not at present direct legal compulsion, but indirect sanctions stemming from malpractice liability.[16] This method of control of drug utilization was probably not envisioned by Congress; however, some current proposals under consideration seek to give such FDA regulations the effect of law.[17] It is not at all surprising that the FDA's proposed rule making on approved uses of drugs has provoked a storm of protest from parts of the medical profession, most notably from the American Medical Association.[18] In this area, the medical profession and the FDA are at odds on one of the more important issues of its type in the history of therapeutic practice.

A major defect of these two methods of control—availability and usage restrictions—as currently employed in the U.S. is that they apply without distinction to all physicians in the country. For example, a cardiologist at a university hospital is deterred from using beta-blockers in hypertension, and a neurologist was at one time deterred from using carbamazepine for epilepsy to the same extent that a dermatologist would be deterred from the same actions. This is illogical, because some physicians are more expert in certain areas than in others. Furthermore, there are bound to be some who are more expert than the members of the national committee by whose decisions they are governed, particularly in view of the conflict-of-interest rules currently applied to the selection of advisory committee members.

These two methods of control are interrelated: it has been officially proposed that grounds for removal of a drug from the market should include "inappropriate" use by the medical profession—for example, for unlabeled uses or inappropriate dosage.[19]

Alternative methods of influencing drug utilization should be sought that are more responsive to the needs of individual patients than the methods currently relied upon. There are several alternatives. We have already examined compulsory avenues such as the legislative, regulatory and medicolegal constraints. There are non-compulsory avenues such as education, persuasion, example, and encouragement. A wide range of specific measures is available. The physician, who must be the focus of most attempts to influence usage, can be reached through professional channels such as educational efforts and peer review. The patient can be educated and made aware of his responsibilities by several mechanisms, including package inserts, advice from knowledgeable pharmacists, and the efforts of consumer groups. In addition, there is a wide range of third parties that have interest and influence, ranging from government regulatory agencies to government and private insurance programs which pay for drugs.

For any system to have much chance of working, it must offer physicians clear assistance in providing improved medical care for their patients. If the rights and responsibilities of any individual physician are to be curtailed, this should be done in a way that is acceptable to the medical profession; the compensatory benefits should be clearly discernible.

A sensible approach would be to experiment with different types of assistance, guidance, or constraint aimed at the physician in order to determine empirically what is best for the American situation.

The educational process is obviously an important channel for improving drug utilization and has been relatively neglected. It would include the dissemination of meaningful information about drugs from a number of sources, both within and outside the medical profession. In some other countries the government's primary effort is educational and takes the form of publications designed to upgrade the level of drug knowledge of the medical community. In the United States, the AMA in particular has persevered in this area for many years. The FDA should devote more attention to voluntary methods of improving utilization, if only to balance the image created by its efforts in the compulsory areas. It should also support work designed to measure the relative effectiveness of the different forms of influence. Recent FDA moves in this direction are a welcome sign.

Another potential influence that should be explored is that offered by programs of third-party payment for drugs. The New Zealand and the Australian systems described earlier are highly developed examples.[20] The American systems of restrictions on the drugs that are eligible for supply under Medicare and Medicaid are newer and still developing examples, although at present these are aimed mainly at reducing costs. As shown by the New Zealand example, third-party payment is one way in which considerable direction of drug utilization can be achieved without excessively infringing the right of any physician to treat any patient as he thinks best.

This approach can allow a number of avenues to be explored, including approved uses and distinction between specialists. Specialization has generally been accepted by the medical profession in every therapeutic modality except the use of drugs; restriction of certain drugs to particular specialists or prescribing situations has not so far found favor. Third-party channels offer the possibility of creating approved indications without resorting to legal sanctions and without erecting insurmountable barriers to the treatment of patients with special needs. Distinctions can be made between physicians of different specialties or levels of training and continuing education. While such distinctions are generally thought of as unpalatable to American physicians, the principle has been firmly established and accepted in the administration of formularies at American hospitals. The use of third-party payment systems to extend this principle to community-wide use may be one of the more practical and less objectionable methods available.

In the area of therapeutic use of investigational drugs, it would also make sense to recognize some distinction between the use of drugs in hospitals and outside hospitals. The hypotensive actions of diazoxide were well known, and the drug had been investigated in the United States for 10 years before it was approved for use in hypertensive emergencies here in 1973. It is difficult to believe that a decade of clinical investigation was needed to justify the use of one or two injections of this drug in emergency situations in a hospital; indeed, this use of the drug was vindicated within a year or two of its first administration to man. If a drug available abroad is believed to have value, it is not sensible for a government agency to deny that drug to properly qualified specialists in major hospitals in this country. As pointed out earlier, the only conditions needed for the use of such a drug are safety precautions and a scientific approach. This is another example of the strong case for substantially liberalizing the individually sponsored investigative use of new drugs. An alternative approach would be to exempt therapeutic use from IND control altogether. While the current IND system is not at all suited to the therapeutic use of investigational drugs, the regulations could probably be adapted; and there is much to be gained, from the scientific point of view, from keeping therapeutic use within the IND system.

Control over Market Access. Control over access of a drug to the market is a blunt, but nonetheless double-edged sword. The changes we have suggested in this chapter would diminish society's need to rely on this unsuitable weapon. If unmarketed and unapproved drugs are made more accessible to individual physicians and their patients so that therapeutic use can be made of these drugs for justifiable purposes, if monitored release allows useful new drugs to be released to the market earlier, if postmarketing surveillance of all drugs can be intensified with proper feedback to the physicians, and if alternative and acceptable measures can be used to influence the utilization of drugs, then the present key role of control over the access of drugs to the market would lose most of its importance.

Furthermore, if, by means of these alternative pathways, drug usage can be made as rational as possible, the FDA's threat to remove drugs from the market in response to unapproved uses or dosages will be rendered unnecessary.

General Improvements

Declassify drug information. A curious shroud of secrecy surrounds knowledge gained by the pharmaceutical industry about the effects of new drugs on animals and man. This deprives the scientific community of helpful information and shields research from the peer scrutiny that should characterize scientific endeavor. The reason given for such secrecy is protection of trade secrets and competitive positions. It is doubtful, however, whether this purpose is actually achieved. At the time clinical trials begin, the compound and most relevant information about it—short of manufacturing processes—will have had to be fully described to at least parts of the academic community, after which any attempt to maintain watertight security is futile. Nevertheless, there is an exaggerated effort to keep the decision-making process and the information on which decisions are based secret from the scientific community—at least for new drugs.

A classic current example is the issue of the putative carcinogenicity in animals of some of the newer beta-agonist and beta-blocking drugs. No comprehensive account of the facts has ever been presented to the medical and scientific community, and most of the independent people who would have an interest in this topic are aware of no more than the outlines of the issues.

The responsibility for releasing more information clearly lies in the first place with the pharmaceutical industry. At the same time, government should not unnecessarily restrict access to the information which it has.

One should note that the U.S. is not the only country plagued by classification fever. In the British Medicines Act, implemented in 1971, it is stipulated that

> if any person discloses to any other person . . . any information obtained by or furnished to him in pursuance of this Act, he shall, unless the disclosure was made in the performance of his duty, be guilty of an offense . . . [carrying penalties of] a fine not exceeding £400 . . . or to imprisonment for a term not exceeding two years, or to both.

Making information more available should be a first step in opening the whole process of drug development to greater public scrutiny. There is profound ignorance of this process in academic, professional, and government circles, and in the media. Individuals in all these communities should be encouraged to grasp the nature of the drug development process at all levels and the principles on which it is based. DeFelice has made the useful suggestion that major pharmaceutical firms should make available for learning purposes the facts about how some of their prototype drugs were developed, so that the evaluation of the course of a drug from a test tube to the pharmacist's shelf will finally be open to examination and criticism. He has also suggested that residencies should be established for clinical pharmacologist trainees within the industry.[22]

Utilize foreign data. The U.S. should make use of not only foreign data on toxicity, but also foreign data on drug efficacy to overcome the profound ignorance of foreign drugs among American physicians.

Surveillance and general information-gathering operations should routinely extend beyond the confines of the United States. Information about the effect on man of new—or indeed any—drugs is a precious world resource. A national agency that disregards foreign data, or, by creating idiosyncratic standards, effectively excludes foreign data from its purview, gratuitously denies itself the benefits of this resource. Furthermore, by forcing its own medical scientists to duplicate existing data, it tends to lower the intellectual standard of clinical pharmacology in its own country, to raise the risk and cost of drug research, and to suppress the innovative process.

Official FDA policy with regard to overseas experience was, until very recently, remarkably parochial. It was only in September 1973 that the FDA officially proposed changing its policy of ignoring evidence on efficacy obtained overseas. The change was adopted in April 1975. In the preamble to this proposal, it is stated that

> the Food and Drug Administration's (FDA's) access to data produced by drug studies performed outside of the United States has been limited largely to review of the published literature. As a result, in reviewing a New Drug Application (NDA) submitted for approval the agency has relied almost exclusively on clinical investigations performed in the United States even though the new drug regulations (21CFR 130.3 and 130.4) permit inclusion of studies performed outside of this country.[23]

A double standard appears to have existed for interpreting foreign data. It is alleged that in some therapeutic areas FDA policy was to regard all evidence of harm from abroad as acceptable no matter how poor its quality, while no evidence of efficacy or benefit was acceptable no matter how high its quality.

These developments have some bearing on the truth of drug labeling. In October 1972 the FDA stated that "Congress intended the labeling to be a full, complete, honest and accurate appraisal of the important facts that have reliably been proved about the drug."[24] It seems, however, that this principle only applied to data generated within the United States. To what extent the proposed new policy actually will be implemented remains to be seen. The policy of ignoring foreign clinical data on efficacy and of requiring American studies of a drug to begin *ab initio* has been one of the most arrogant notions in the history of drug regulation. The effects of this attitude on the American patient have already been documented. The way in which these ideas came into being and held sway for so long should be carefully examined.

Advisory committees. The recent FDA trend to rely more on advisory committees is a hopeful sign; the curious belief, held until recently, that drug review could and should be an internal operation of the regulatory agency was an almost uniquely American phenomenon.

There is a strong need for the FDA to establish its scientific expertise and credibility by using the best resources of talent in the nation. It is also desirable for scientific decisions to be separated from the regulatory function of the FDA. Advisory committees selected from the academic and professional communities are an obvious way to do this, and it is encouraging to observe the progress that is being made in this area.

It is disturbing to note that this sensible trend within the FDA has been criticized by an overseeing committee of the House of Representatives.[25] While excessive use of advisory committees is generally to be deplored in any branch of government, it should be clearly understood that in the area of drugs, advisory committees are needed on an increasingly large scale because of the exceptionally technical nature of the material and because of the difficulty of implementing law in a manner that makes sense both scientifically and medically.

Some issues about the use of advisory committees remain unresolved: On whose behalf are they making decisions and what is the legal status of the advice they give? It should be understood that the ultimate function of any such committee, and indeed of the regulatory agency itself, is to preempt decision making that would otherwise fall to patients and their physicians. Any third parties which become involved should be viewed as servants of the patient and the physician rather than as masters. Who should select the members and what safeguards should there be to ensure that a committee is competent to deal with the issues presented to it? Conspicuous problems have arisen recently due to inappropriately selected committees.

A peculiarity of the American system that deserves close scrutiny is the fact that major therapeutic decisions are increasingly being made in the courts. Recent court actions over the use of tolbutamide for diabetes and betahistine for Menière's disease are signs of a system that is using legal arguments as a substitute for scientific facts. Judging from their recent performance, courts seem to be the least appropriate arbiters of complex questions of medical science and practice. The problem here is that the scientific answers are at present indeterminate; no need for a legal solution would exist if the scientific issues were unequivocal. Within the framework of due process, the aim should be to deal with scientific and medical issues on their scientific and medical merits rather than on legal ones.

Measured benefits versus risks. Among the defects in our current methods of making decisions on safety and efficacy is the lack of operational definitions and an attendant lack of data on which to operate. This is especially true of data on the benefits drugs produce.

Since thalidomide, philosophies have tended towards the extreme interpretation of *primum non nocere* at the expense of "first do some good for the patient." All decisions about risk and benefit are currently severely hampered by the paucity of data on the benefits drugs produce under conditions of actual use; imbalanced decisions result when inadequate data on benefit are weighed against the voluminous, if often scientifically questionable, data available on hazards.

There is thus a great need to develop methodology for measuring benefit in its economic and social as well as medical forms. It would be desirable to ensure that surveillance plans devote as much effort to measuring benefits as to detecting hazards. This obvious and important point has not yet penetrated far into regulatory consciousness. As recently as May 16, 1973, Phase IV studies were defined within the FDA's Biometric and Epidemiological Methodology Advisory Committee exclusively in terms of the assessment of drug safety. There was no reference to any effects of drugs other than harmful ones.[26]

Economic measures of benefit and cost form a potent but—at least in medical analyses—neglected approach.[27] Most considerations are addressed only to the reduction of drug prices. Since, however, the cost of drug therapy is less than 10 percent of total health-care costs, even large reductions in expenditure on drugs can have but minor impact on the total cost of health care. In other ways, however, drugs are one of the few approaches in medicine that can produce savings—for example, by reducing hospitalization, as in infectious disease and mental illness.

The public interest. Despite all that has been said and written about the pharmaceutical industry, little or no attention has been given to defining precisely where the public interest lies in the process of drug development and utilization. There is no comprehensive, balanced analysis of what society should require from physicians, government, and the pharmaceutical industry, nor of how each sector should best meet those needs. In most discussions, society's needs are taken to be implicit and obvious. On the contrary, these needs are not at all obvious; they involve wider issues than medical ones, and some of the needs are conflicting. A comprehensive analysis is needed in order to put all components into perspective. Consumer groups have so far been of no help to the patient who has a disease for which currently available therapy is imperfect in efficacy or safety or nonexistent. In ignoring such needs and in pursuing policies that will result in slowing the process of drug development, consumer groups are acting against the interest of sick patients.

The public economic interest involves the total cost of medical care, and legislation should be based on more comprehensive economic analyses than those available to date. In the medical area, we need to learn how to ensure the most appropriate, effective and safe use of existing drugs, how to integrate drugs and other modalities in a total therapeutic armamentarium, and how to develop better drugs.

Positive legislation and regulation. For too long in the United States, the function of the law and of the FDA has been conceived as protecting the public from harm by keeping new and potentially dangerous drugs off the market. We have shown that this narrowly negative view is in many ways unfortunate. An equally important positive function should be to encourage the development and wise use of better drugs.

Another trend, seen clearly in the hearings on propranolol, has been to demand excessive requirements for proof of efficacy before a drug or a new use is approved. Since the perfect drug study has yet to be performed, grounds can always be found for faulting individual studies. This is an area in which more credence could be given to the ability of physicians and patients to judge a drug's efficacy in particular cases.

Despite recent improvements in its attitude, one still hears the view that the FDA cannot be blamed for delaying the introduction of an admittedly useful new drug into the United States if the NDA was submitted later here than abroad. This argument has been used recently in the case of carbenoxolone, rifampin, and cromolyn sodium.[28] This argument fails to recognize that a positive approach is possible. If a useful new drug of proven merit exists anywhere in the world, it should be the duty of the FDA to know about that drug and, if not to ensure that it is made available to American patients who need it, then at least not to hinder their access. Whether this could be achieved by liberalizing the private IND process, or whether it would require more radical measures, needs to be determined. In any case, this argument also overlooks the fact that the greater data requirements for an NDA in the U.S. in themselves delay filing until data are accumulated from American clinical trials.

Recent congressional criticism [29] of the FDA's welcomed new policies give little cause for optimism. If this reaction persists, we face the beginning of a new dark age of American therapeutics before we have fully emerged from the previous one.

CHAPTER XIV

CONCLUSIONS

It is unlikely that the present state of drug development and utilization was that intended by Congress when the relevant laws were enacted. This fact is not generally perceived. There is also little general awareness of what the public policy issues are and what Congress should be trying to achieve in this area.

In the face of this lack of understanding, the medical profession cannot effectively counter groups who argue that patients would be better served if physicians had less autonomy in drug utilization and third parties had more control. Likewise, government may continue to assume that its particular style of regulating drug development over the past decade has produced the most public benefit for the least harm. And the pharmaceutical industry cannot prove that society would be any worse off if industry's research on new drugs were slowed by official constraints on drug profitability and thereby on the research process. It is encouraging to observe that the latter dilemma has at least been discussed at recent congressional hearings. However, there is an obvious need to define clearly the public interest in all these areas and to develop techniques for measuring how this interest is being fulfilled.

It is particularly necessary to define the importance of research into the discovery and development of better drugs and to examine how legislative and regulatory policies affect such research activity. There is already evidence to suggest that the research and development performance of the pharmaceutical industry in the United States is being handicapped relative to the industry abroad; this is clearly an area that needs prompt research to define the contribution, if any, of regulatory factors. In our opinion, the public interest would be well served by policies designed to stimulate the development and introduction of better medicines. It would be a historic and entirely feasible step if government agencies, including the FDA, were given formal mandates to do this.

The growing involvement of third parties in the relationship between physician and patient may represent the most significant development in the modern history of medical practice. Common sense would suggest that such participation should reflect planned and coordinated efforts of the medical professions, the sciences, and the agencies of society at large, with research to determine the best form of involvement. At present, however, third-party participation arises as an incidental and unforeseen by-product of activities in other areas. These trends deserve careful study. It is doubtful whether enough information exists at present to evaluate the overall benefits and losses that accrue to a society when fundamental decision-making power in the management of individual patients is removed from the patient's physician and assumed by third parties. The issue is a novel one historically. There has been little formal study of the effects of either such policies in general or one particular aspect of them, namely, the assumption that to minimize toxicity is to maximize benefit. Nevertheless, this principle has in the past been acted on extensively in the United States, with generally tacit acceptance by the medical profession. There is a growing risk that it may again come to be implemented rigidly. As Dunlop [1] has pointed out, it is paradoxical that, in terms of drug therapeutics, the British practitioner under socialized medicine is more free to exercise his professional judgment than is his American counterpart in an ostensibly less restrictive system.

The Food and Drug Administration in the United States has been the first regulatory agency to identify many of these policy conflicts and to propose formal regulatory solutions; they deserve credit for identifying the issues. It is clear, however, that not everyone agrees with the solutions proposed and that there has so far been inadequate response to these important proposals by the academic and professional medical communities.

If one compares the American with the British approach to these problems, some fundamental differences emerge. In the case of new drugs, or new uses for existing drugs, it is widely accepted in the U.S. that it is proper for a regulatory agency to make therapeutic risk-benefit decisions on behalf of all physicians and all patients. In Britain, on the other hand, the regulatory agency has so far been content to leave more of these decisions to individual physicians; it has concentrated on educational rather than regulatory pressure to ensure the best possible prescribing. Without empirical study, one cannot be certain which of these approaches is best, either for the welfare of individual patients or for society as a whole. The most desirable approach may differ in two countries so disparate in size, philosophy and approach to the provision of medical care. This is an issue on which evidence could be obtained. The lack of attention to this problem from either the medical profession or the academic community is surprising. The implications of this trend are obviously not fully appreciated.

As we have shown, the situation is fluid. Over the past two years developments have occurred in the U.S. that would have seemed inconceivable even a year or two ago. The regulatory process has become the object of the renewed interest and concern of the broad medical community, and new government administrators have appeared with a better grasp of the scientific and medical problems involved.

These hopeful developments are evidence that the system can produce and accept informed criticism; but the gains are fragile and hard won, and there is pressure for a return to the old ways. We earnestly hope, in the interest of sick patients everywhere, that such progress will be fostered.

Controls on Medical Practice

For a number of reasons, including the fact that their production and use is an easily identifiable sector of medical practice, therapeutic drugs have so far borne the brunt of attention from third parties. These trends are, however, already extending into other areas of medicine, as seen for example in the creation of professional standards review organizations. Drug control is a paradigm of third-party influences on medical practice; the medical profession has lost most of the initiative it once had in the process of drug development and is now losing control of the way drugs are utilized. It is remarkable that the results of these influences have been so little studied that we cannot yet tell whether the patient is better or worse off as a result of them.

Society has found it unexpectedly easy to regulate the development of new drugs. Some attention should now be devoted to ascertaining the precise effects of the present controls and to ensuring that they are directed entirely towards the patients' interests—which will, in turn, require an adequate understanding of those interests.

Role of the FDA

One cannot accurately evaluate or compare regulatory, industrial and other factors in the complex set of influences that have created the distinctive features of current American therapeutics. Nevertheless, legislative and regulatory policies are obviously important causes. The marked changes of the past year are largely a result of improved regulatory policies towards the introduction of new drugs. While this is heartening evidence of response to informed criticism and suggestions, it is also evidence that room for improvement indeed existed and that the previous state of affairs could have been the result of earlier regulatory policies.

The FDA's role in the drug innovation process is complex. The same policies that contributed, directly or indirectly, to the delay in new drug approvals contributed also to the enormous improvement in the standard of investigation of new drugs in both industry and academia. One must also acknowledge that delay of drug approval acts as insurance against hazards subsequently discovered in other countries; the debate concerns the relative gains and losses of that approach.

Furthermore, it should be recognized that, while the FDA has no mandate to direct the practice of medicine, it is the express purpose of some governmental bodies, such as other parts of HEW and the Drug Enforcement Agency, to change the way medicine is practiced. Thus, in comparison with other sources of influence, it is conceivable that the FDA could emerge as a protector of the status quo in medical practice rather than the agent of change many people currently consider it.

Legislation as Experimentation

Medicine has important lessons to learn from the bold American actions taken over the past twelve years to tighten the regulation of drugs and therapeutics. Like the drugs they set out to control, the 1962 laws and their regulatory implementation have had mixed results.[2] Indeed, if judged by the same standards they themselves set for drugs, the 1962 laws could not be approved because no evidence of their safety or efficacy exists: they were implemented in a scientifically uncontrolled manner, and no measures of their effects were even sought. We are only now beginning to evaluate in retrospect the effects of the changes that began in 1962, and it is doubtful whether their full impact can ever be known.

The fundamental point, generally unrecognized, is that any legislative or regulatory intervention is an experiment which deserves careful planning of its design and evaluation.[3] We are now at the threshold of larger and bolder legislative and regulatory experiments that affect not only drugs but also the broader fabric of medical practice. We should at the very least acknowledge the experimental nature of these new policies and act accordingly. Their implementation must be designed as the experiment it is—with valid controls and systems for measuring the results set up in advance. Only in this way can the impact of new legislation and regulation be ascertained and the greatest possible benefits for society realized.

APPENDIX

DEFINITION OF "SUBSTANTIAL EVIDENCE"

Section 505(d) of the Federal Food, Drug and Cosmetic Act, as amended, 1972, reads as follows:

As used in this subsection and subsection (e), the term "substantial evidence" means evidence consisting of adequate and well-controlled investigations, including clinical investigations, by experts qualified by scientific training and experience to evaluate the effectiveness of the drug involved, on the basis of which it could fairly and responsibly be concluded by such experts that the drug will have the effect it purports or is represented to have under the conditions of use prescribed, recommended, or suggested in the labeling or proposed labeling thereof.

Requirements for Proof of Drug Efficacy

Part 130.12 of the New Drug Regulations amendment of May 8, 1970, as published in the *Federal Register,* May 8, 1970, p. 7250, includes the following as grounds on which the FDA commissioner shall refuse to approve a New Drug Application:

(5) (i) Evaluated on the basis of information submitted as part of the application and any other information before the Food and Drug Administration with respect to such drug, there is lack of substantial evidence consisting of adequate and well-controlled investigations, including clinical investigations, by experts qualified by scientific training and experience to evaluate the effectiveness of the drug involved, on the basis of which it could fairly and responsibly be concluded by such experts that the drug will have the effect it purports

or is represented to have under the conditions of use prescribed, recommended, or suggested in the proposed labeling.

[The amendment then goes on to state:]

(ii) The following principles have been developed over a period of years and are recognized by the scientific community as the essentials of adequate and well-controlled clinical investigations. They provide the basis for the determination whether there is "substantial evidence" to support the claims of effectiveness for "new drugs" and antibiotic drugs.

(a) The plan or protocol for the study and the report of the results of the effectiveness study must include the following:

(1) A clear statement of the objectives of the study.

(2) A method of selection of the subjects that—

(i) Provides adequate assurance that they are suitable for the purposes of the study, diagnostic criteria of the condition to be treated or diagnosed, confirmatory laboratory tests where appropriate, and, in the case of prophylactic agents, evidence of susceptibility and exposure to the condition against which prophylaxis is desired.

(ii) Assigns the subjects to test groups in such a way as to minimize bias.

(iii) Assures comparability in test and control groups of pertinent variables, such as age, sex, severity, or duration of disease, and use of drugs other than the test drugs.

(3) Explains the methods of observation and recording of results, including the variables measured, quantitation, assessment of any subjective response, and steps taken to minimize bias on the part of the subject and observer.

(4) Provides a comparison of the results of treatment or diagnosis with a control in such a fashion as to permit quantitative evaluation. The precise nature of the control must be stated and an explanation given of the methods used to minimize bias on the part of the observers and the analysts of the data. Level and methods of "blinding," if used, are to be documented. Generally, four types of comparison are recognized:

(i) No treatment: Where objective measurements of effectiveness are available and placebo effect is negligible, comparison of the objective results in comparable groups of treated and untreated patients.

(ii) Placebo control: Comparison of the results of use of the new drug entity with an inactive preparation designed to resemble the test drug as far as possible.

(iii) Active treatment control: An effective regimen of therapy may be used for comparison, e.g., where the condition treated is such that no treatment or administration of a placebo would be contrary to the interest of the patient.

(iv) Historical control: In certain circumstances, such as those involving diseases with high and predictable mortality (acute leukemia of childhood), with signs and symptoms of predictable duration or severity (fever in certain infections), or, in case of prophylaxis, where morbidity is predictable, the results of use of a new drug entity may be compared quantitatively with prior experience historically derived from the adequately documented natural history of the disease or condition in comparable patients or populations with no treatment or with a regimen (therapeutic, diagnostic, prophylactic) the effectiveness of which is established.

(5) A summary of the methods of analysis and an evaluation of data derived from the study, including any appropriate statistical methods.

Provided, however, That any of the above criteria may be waived in whole or in part, either prior to the investigation or in the evaluation of a completed study, by the Director of the Bureau of Drugs with respect to a specific clinical investigation; a petition for such a waiver may be filed by any person who would be adversely affected by the application of the criteria to a particular clinical investigation; the petition should show that some or all of the criteria are not reasonably applicable to the investigation and that alternative procedures can be, or have been, followed, the results of which will or have yielded data that can and should be accepted as substantial evidence of the drug's effectiveness. A petition for a waiver shall set forth clearly and concisely the specific provision or provisions in the criteria from which waiver is sought, why the criteria are not reasonably applicable to the particular clinical investigation, what alternative procedures, if any, are to be, or have been, employed, what results have been obtained, and the basis on which it can be, or has been, concluded that the clinical investigation will or has yielded substantial evidence of effectiveness, notwithstanding nonconformance with the criteria for which waiver is requested.

(b) For such an investigation to be considered adequate for approval of a new drug, it is required that the test drug be standardized as to identity, strength, quality, purity, and dosage form to give significance to the results of the investigation.

(c) Uncontrolled studies or partially controlled studies are not acceptable as the sole basis for the approval of claims of effectiveness. Such studies, carefully conducted and documented, may provide corroborative support of well-controlled studies regarding efficacy and may yield valuable data regarding safety of the test drug.

Such studies will be considered on their merits in the light of the principles listed here, with the exception of the requirement for the comparison of the treated subjects with controls. Isolated case reports, random experience, and reports lacking the details which permit scientific evaluation will not be considered.

NOTES

NOTES TO CHAPTER I

[1] A. Trousseau, *Clinique medicale de l'Hotel-Dieu de Paris* (Paris: Bailliere, 1877), vol. 1, p. 3.

[2] By the authority of the Medical Societies and Colleges, *Pharmacopoeia of the United States of America* (Boston: Wells and Lilly for Charles Ever, December 1820).

[3] American Medical Association, House of Delegates, "Draft Resolutions 58, 59, 60, 75, 85, 90, and substitute resolution 58," 1973, p. 17.

[4] V. A. Kleinfeld, "Commentary of Part IV, Federal Regulation," in *Safeguarding the Public*, ed. J. B. Blake (Baltimore: The Johns Hopkins Press, 1970), p. 182.

NOTES TO CHAPTER II

[1] E. I. Goldenthal, "Current Views on Safety Evaluation of Drugs," *Food and Drug Administration Papers*, May 1968, p. 13.

[2] J. G. Wilson, "Teratogeny in Nonhuman Primates," in *Proceedings of the Conference on Nonhuman Toxicology, June 12-14, 1966* (Washington, D. C.: Government Printing Office, 1966).

[3] World Health Organization, "Principles for the Testing and Evaluation of Drugs for Carcinogenicity," *World Health Organization Technical Reports*, series no. 426 (1969).

[4] Committee on Problems of Drug Safety of the Drug Research Board, NAS-NRC, "Application of Metabolic Data to the Evaluation of Drugs," *Clinical Pharmacology and Therapeutics*, vol. 10 (1969), pp. 607-34.

[5] *FDA Papers*, September 1969.

[6] Pharmaceutical Manufacturers Association, Research and Development Sections, report of an ad hoc committee, mimeo., 1970; personal communication.

NOTES TO CHAPTER III

[1] C. Anello, "FDA Principles in Clinical Investigations," *Food and Drug Administration Papers*, June 1970, pp. 14-24.

[2] Department of Health, Education and Welfare, Food and Drug Administration, "New Drug Regulations under the Federal Food, Drug, and Cosmetic Act," *Federal Register*, vol. 35, no. 90 (May 8, 1970), pp. 7250-53.

[3] National Academy of Science, *Drug Efficacy Study, Final Report to the Commissioner of Food and Drugs* (Washington, D. C., 1969).

[4] M. Reidenberg and D. Lowenthal, "Adverse Nondrug Reactions," *New England Journal of Medicine*, vol. 279 (1968), p. 678.

[5] Subcommittee on the National Halothane Study, Committee on Anesthesia, NAS-NRC, "Summary of the National Halothane Study," *Journal of the American Medical Association*, vol. 197 (1966), pp. 775-88.

[6] C. A. Bunde and H. M. Leyland, "A Controlled Retrospective Survey in Evaluation of Teratogenicity," *Journal of New Drugs*, vol. 5 (1965), pp. 193-98.

[7] J. H. Gaddum, "Clinical Pharmacology," Walter Ernest Dixon Memorial Lecture, *Proceedings of the Royal Society of Medicine*, vol. 47 (1954), pp. 195-204.

[8] L. Lasagna and P. Meier, "Experimental Design and Statistical Problems," in *Clinical Evaluation of New Drugs*, ed. S. O. Waife and A. P. Shapiro (New York: Hoeber-Harper, 1959), pp. 37-60.

[9] A. Feinstein, "An Analytic Appraisal of the University Group Diabetes Program (UGDP) Study," *Clinical Pharmacology and Therapeutics*, vol. 12 (1971), pp. 167-91.

[10] H. S. Mathisen, H. Loken, D. Brox, and O. Stenbaek, "The Prognosis in Long-Term Treated and 'Untreated' Essential Hypertension," *Acta Medica Scandinavica*, vol. 185 (1969), pp. 253-58.

[11] R. Lovell and R. Prineas, "Trends in Prescribing Hypotensive Drugs and in Mortality from Stroke in Australia," *Medical Journal of Australia*, vol. 2 (1971), p. 557.

[12] Sam Peltzman, *Regulation of Pharmaceutical Innovation: The 1962 Amendments* (Washington, D. C.: American Enterprise Institute, 1974), p. 45.

NOTES TO CHAPTER IV

[1] F. J. Ingelfinger, A. S. Relman, and M. Finland, eds., *Controversy in Internal Medicine* (Philadelphia: W. B. Saunders, 1966).

NOTES TO CHAPTER V

[1] Peltzman, *Regulation of Pharmaceutical Innovation*, pp. 10-11.

[2] B. B. Bloom, "The Rate of Contemporary Drug Discovery," in *Advances in Chemistry*, series no. 108 (Washington, D. C.: American Chemical Society, 1971), pp. 176-84.

[3] H. A. Clymer, "The Changing Costs and Risks of Pharmaceutical Innovation," in *The Economics of Drug Innovation*, ed. J. D. Cooper (Washington, D. C.: The American University, 1970), pp. 109-38.

[4] V. A. Mund, "The Return on Investment of the Innovative Pharmaceutical Firm," in ibid., pp. 125-138.

[5] E. H. Mansfield, "Discussion by the Panel," in ibid., pp. 149-51.

[6] C. Djerassi, "Birth Control after 1984," *Science*, vol. 168 (1970), pp. 941-45.

NOTES TO CHAPTER VII

[1] J. Curran, unpublished data supplied by Pfizer, Inc., 235 East 42nd Street, New York, New York, 1971, 1972; Paul de Haen, *Watchlist* (New York: Paul de Haen, Inc., 1971); J. A. Flanders, "Effects of Regulatory Agency Activities on the Rate of New Drug Introductions 1966-71: Some Preliminary Observations," mimeo. (Washington, D. C.: Pharmaceutical Manufacturers Association, 1972).

[2] Paul de Haen, *Non-Proprietary Name Index* (New York: Paul de Haen, Inc., 1971), vol. 18.

[3] *British Pharmaceutical Index* (London: Intercontinental Medical Statistics, Ltd., 1971).

[4] K. H. Beyer, "What Pharmacology Is All About," *The Pharmacologist*, vol. 13 (1971), pp. 129-33; A. Feinstein, "Clinical Biostatistics IX. How Do We Measure 'Safety' and 'Efficacy'?" *Clinical Pharmacology and Therapeutics*, vol. 12 (1971), pp. 544-58.

[5] The Coronary Drug Project Research Group, "Clofibrate and Niacin in Coronary Heart Disease," *Journal of the American Medical Association*, vol. 231 (1975), pp. 360-81.

[6] Peltzman, *Regulation of Pharmaceutical Innovation.*

[7] Ayerst Laboratories, "INDERAL" Brand of Propranolol Hydrochloride, New York, December 1967, package insert.

[8] "A New Approach to the Treatment of Hypertension," *Lancet*, vol. 2 (1970), p. 85; F. O. Simpson and H. J. Waal-Manning, "Hypertension and Beta-Adrenergic Blockade," in *Symposium on Beta-Adrenergic Blockade* (Sydney: Sandoz, 1970); R. Zacest, E. Gilmore, and J. Koch-Weser, "Treatment of Essential Hypertension with Combined Vasodilation and Beta-Adrenergic Blockade," *New England Journal of Medicine*, vol. 286 (1972), pp. 617-22; F. J. Zacharias, "Propranolol in Hypertension: A Five-Year Study," *Postgraduate Medical Journal*, vol. 47 supplementary (January 1971), pp. 75-79.

[9] American Medical Association, *AMA Drug Evaluations* (Chicago, 1971).

[10] T. Killip, "Ischemic Heart Disease," in *Cecil-Loeb Textbook of Medicine*, ed. P. Beeson and W. McDermott (Philadelphia: W. B. Saunders Co., 1971), pp. 1016-39.

[11] "Lidocaine (Xylocaine) as an Antiarrhythmic Agent," *Medical Letter*, vol. 13 (1971), pp. 1-2.

[12] C. F. George, R. E. Nagle, and B. L. Pentecost, "Practolol in Treatment of Angina Pectoris: A Double-Blind Trial," *British Medical Journal*, vol. 2 (1970), pp. 402-4.

[13] Simpson and Waal-Manning, "Hypertension and Beta-Adrenergic Blockade"; B. N. C. Prichard, A. J. Boakes and G. Day, "Practolol in the Treatment of Hypertension," *Postgraduate Medical Journal*, vol. 47 supplementary (1971), pp. 84-92.

[14] J. Vohra, J. Dowling, and G. Sloman, "Practolol (ICI 50171), A Beta-Adrenergic Receptor Blocking Agent, in the Management of Cardiac Arrhythmias," *Medical Journal of Australia*, vol. 2 (1970), pp. 228-31.

[15] D. F. Wilson, O. F. Watson, J. S. Peel, and A. S. Turner, "Trasicor in Angina: A Double-Blind Trial," *British Medical Journal*, vol. 2 (1969), pp. 155-57.

[16] Simpson and Waal-Manning, "Hypertension and Beta-Adrenergic Blockade."

[17] D. G. Gibson, "Haemodynamic Effects of Practolol," *Postgraduate Medical Journal*, vol. 47 supplementary (January 1971), pp. 16-21; A. Pitt and S. T. Anderson, "A Comparison of the Effects of Trasicor (Oxprenolol) and Inderal (Propranolol) on Left Ventricular Myocardial Function," *Medical Journal of Australia*, vol. 1 (1970), pp. 1089-93.

[18] H. M. Beumer, "Local Effects of Beta-Adrenergic Blocking Drugs in Histamine Sensitive Asthmatics," *Pharmacologia Clinica*, vol. 1 (1969), pp. 171-73.

[19] Ayerst Laboratories, package insert.

[20] W. M. Wardell, "Fluroxene and the Penicillin Lesson," *Anesthesiology*, vol. 38 (1973), pp. 309-12.

[21] S. Ferebee, "Controlled Chemoprophylaxis Trials in Tuberculosis," *Advances in Tuberculosis Research*, vol. 17 (1970), pp. 28-186.

[22] M. Rustia and P. Shubik, "Induction of Lung Tumours and Malignant Lymphomas in Mice by Metronidazole," *Journal of the National Cancer Institute*, vol. 48 (1972), pp. 721-29.

[23] S. Epstein, J. Andrea, S. Joshi and N. Mantel, "Hepatocarcinogenicity of Griseofulvin Following Parenteral Administration to Infant Mice," *Cancer Research*, vol. 27 (1967), pp. 1900-6.

[24] B. N. C. Prichard, A. W. Johnston, I. D. Hill, and M. L. Rosenheim, "Bethanidine, Guanethidine and Methyldopa in Treatment of Hypertension: A Within-Patient Comparison," *British Medical Journal*, vol. 1 (1968), pp. 135-44.

[25] F. O. Simpson, "Combination Antihypertensive Therapy," *International Cardiology*, vol. 2 (1970), p. 3; and 'Cardiovascular Clinics," pp. 38-54.

[26] G. E. Bauer, "Debrisoquine: A Five-Year Study of a New Hypotensive Agent," *Medical Journal of Australia*, vol. 2 (1970), p. 911; A. Heffernan, A. Carty, K. O'Malley, and J. Bugler, "A Within-Patient Comparison of Debrisoquine and Methyldopa in Hypertension," *British Medical Journal*, vol. 1 (1971), pp. 75-78.

[27] J. V. Hodge, "Guanoclor as an Antihypertensive Drug," *British Medical Journal*, vol. 2 (1966), pp. 981-84; T. D. V. Lawrie, A. R. Lorimer, S. G. McAlpine, and H. Reinert, "Clinical Trial and Pharmacological Study of Compound 1029 (Vatensol)," *British Medical Journal*, vol. 1 (1964), pp. 402-6; W. S. Peart and M. T. MacMahon, "Clinical Trial of 2-guanidinomethyl (1,4)-benzodioxan (Compound 1003)," *British Medical Journal*, vol. 1 (1964), pp. 398-402.

[28] Lawrie et al., "Clinical Trial," pp. 402-6; G. Persson, B. Ekwall, and C. Furst, "A Clinical Trial of Guanoxan (Envacar) in Hypertension Resistant to Common Drugs," *Acta Medica Scandinavica*, vol. 182 (1967), pp. 567-74.

[29] H. E. Simmons, Statement before the Subcommittee on Monopoly, Senate Select Committee on Small Business, February 5, 1973 (Food and Drug Administration typescript).

[30] *British Pharmaceutical Index*, 1971.

[31] U.S. Food and Drug Administration, "Notice of the Opportunity for a Hearing on the Proposal to Withdraw Approval of New Drug Applications (Mebutamate Tablets—Wallace Pharmaceuticals)," *Federal Register*, vol. 38, no. 33 (1973), pp. 4683-84.

[32] S. W. Hoobler and E. Sagastume, "Clonidine Hydrochloride in the Treatment of Hypertension," *American Journal of Cardiology*, vol. 28 (1971), pp. 67-73; G. Onesti, K. D. Bock, V. Heimsoth, K. E. Kim, and P. Merguet, "Clonidine: A New Antihypertensive Agent," *American Journal of Cardiology*, vol. 28 (1971), pp. 74-83; B. K. Yeh, A. Nantel, and L. I. Goldberg, "Antihypertensive Effect of Clonidine," *Archives of Internal Medicine*, vol. 127 (1971), pp. 233-37.

[33] Hoobler and Sagastume, "Clonidine Hydrochloride," pp. 67-73; Yeh et al., "Antihypertensive Effect," pp. 233-37.

[34] Onesti et al., "Clonidine," pp. 74-83.

[35] J. Shafar, E. R. Tallett, and P. A. Knowlson, "Evaluation of Clonidine in Prophylaxis of Migraine," *Lancet*, vol. 1 (1972), pp. 403-7.

[36] O. L. Wade, *Adverse Reactions to Drugs* (London: William Heinemann Medical Books, Ltd., 1970), pp. 37-40.

[37] D. Cahal, "Jaundice and Cardivix," *British Medical Journal*, vol. 2 (1964), p. 882; J. Valentine, J. Cox, and G. Devey, "Jaundice and Cardivix," *British Medical Journal*, vol. 2 (1964), p. 882.

[38] J. Condemi, "Cromolyn Treatment of Asthma," *Journal of the American Medical Association*, vol. 216 (1971), p. 1454-58; C. Falliers, "Cromolyn Sodium (Disodium Cromoglycate)," *Journal of Allergy*, vol. 47 (1971), pp. 298-305; J. Howell, "The Present Status of Sodium Cromoglycate," *The Practitioner*, vol. 208 (1972), pp. 750-56.

[39] Howell, "The Present Status of Sodium Cromoglycate," pp. 750-56; E. Holopainen, A. Backman, and O. Salo, "Effect of Disodium Cromoglycate on Seasonal Allergic Rhinitis," *Lancet*, vol. 1 (1971), pp. 55-57.

[40] R. T. Brittain, "A Comparison of the Pharmacology of Salbutamol with that of Isoprenaline, Orciprenaline and Trimetoquinol," *Postgraduate Medical Journal*, vol. 47 supplementary (March 1971), pp. 11-16; V. Cullum, J. Farmer, D. Jack, and G. Levy, "Salbutamol: A New, Selective β-Adrenoreceptive Receptor Stimulant," *British Journal of Pharmacology*, vol. 35 (1969), pp. 141-51; C. M. Fletcher, H. Herxheimer, J. B. L. Howell, A. Lewis, and D. Jack, "Salbutamol: An International Symposium," *Postgraduate Medical Journal*, vol. 47 supplementary (1971); H. Formgren, "A Clinical Comparison of the Effect of Oral Terbutaline and Orciprenaline," *Scandinavian Journal of Respiratory Diseases*, vol. 51 (1970), pp. 195-202.

[41] B. Cohen, "Studies with Isoetharine I. The Ventilatory Effects of Aerosol and Oral Forms," *Journal of Asthma Research*, vol. 4 (1967), pp. 209-18, and

"Studies with Isoetharine II. Cardiovascular Effects in Hypertensive Patients with Expiratory Air Flow Disorders," pp. 259-67.

[42] P. Heaf, "Deaths in Asthma: A Therapeutic Misadventure?" *British Medical Bulletin*, vol. 26 (1970), pp. 245-47.

[43] M. Conolly, D. Davies, C. Dollery, and C. George, "Resistance to β-Adrenoceptor," *British Journal of Pharmacology*, vol. 43 (1971), pp. 389-402.

[44] P. Stolley, "Asthma Mortality," *American Review of Respiratory Disease*, vol. 105 (1972), pp. 883-90.

[45] L. Garrod, "Trimethoprim: Its Possible Place in Therapy," *Drugs*, vol. 1 (1971), pp. 3-6.

[46] W. M. Wardell, "Introduction of New Therapeutic Drugs in the United States and Great Britain: An International Comparison," *Clinical Pharmacology and Therapeutics*, vol. 14 (1973), pp. 773-90, and "British Usage and American Awareness of Some New Therapeutic Drugs," pp. 1022-34.

[47] R. Cooper and M. Wald, "Successful Treatment of Proteus Septicaemia with a New Drug, Trimethoprim," *Medical Journal of Australia*, vol. 2 (1964), pp. 93-96; E. Noall, H. Sewards, and P. Waterworth, "Successful Treatment of a Case of Proteus Septicaemia," *British Medical Journal*, vol. 2 (1962), pp. 1101-2.

[48] J. Darrell, L. Garrod, and P. Waterworth, "Trimethoprim: Laboratory and Clinical Studies," *Journal of Clinical Pathology*, vol. 21 (1968), pp. 202-9.

[49] A. G. Baikie, C. B. Macdonald, and G. R. Mundy, "Systemic Nocardiosis Treated with Trimethoprim and Sulphamethoxazole," *Lancet*, vol. 2 (1970), p. 261.

[50] American Medical Association, *AMA Drug Evaluations*, 1971.

[51] Beeson and McDermott, eds., *Cecil-Loeb Textbook of Medicine*.

[52] W. Modell, ed., *Drugs of Choice 1972-1973* (St. Louis: C. V. Mosby Company, 1972).

[53] L. Q. Garrod and F. O'Grady, *Antibiotic and Chemotherapy*, 3rd ed. (London: Churchill Livingstone, 1971).

[54] K. Jensen and H. Lassen, "Combined Treatment with Antibacterial Chemotherapeutic Agents in Staphylococcal Infections," *Quarterly Journal of Medicine* (new series), vol. 38 (1969), pp. 91-106.

[55] N. Blockey and T. McAllister, "Antibiotics in Acute Osteomyelitis in Children," *Journal of Bone and Joint Surgery*, vol. 54B (1972), pp. 299-309; D. Rowling, "Further Experience in the Management of Chronic Osteomyelitis," *Journal of Bone and Joint Surgery*, vol. 52B (1970), pp. 302-7.

[56] National Center for Health Statistics, Department of Health, Education and Welfare, *Vital Statistics of the United States 1968* (Rockville, Md., 1971), vol. 2, part B.

[57] Peltzman, *Regulation of Pharmaceutical Innovation*, p. 62.

[58] A. Shapiro and E. Shapiro, "Treatment of Gilles de la Tourette's Syndrome with Haloperidol," *British Journal of Psychiatry*, vol. 114 (1968), pp. 345-50.

[59] Wardell, "Introduction of New Therapeutic Drugs," p. 783.

[60] M. Dalby, "Antiepileptic and Psychotropic Effect of Carbamazepine (Tegretol) in the Treatment of Psychomotor Epilepsy," *Epilepsia*, vol. 12 (1971), pp. 325-34; W. E. Pryse-Phillips and P. M. Jeavons, "Effect of Carbamazepine on the Electroencephalograph and Ward Behaviour of Patients with Chronic Epilepsy," *Epilepsia*, vol. 11 (1970), pp. 263-73.

[61] E. Woodward, "Clinical Experience with Fenfluramine in the United States," in *International Symposium on Amphetamines and Related Compounds*, ed. E. Costa and S. Garattini (New York: Raven Press, 1970), pp. 685-91.

[62] O. Follows, "A Comparative Trial of Fenfluramine and Diethylpropion in Obese, Hypertensive Patients," *British Journal of Clinical Practice*, vol. 25 (1971), pp. 236-38.

[63] S. Lewis, I. Oswald, and D. Dunleavy, "Chronic Fenfluramine Administration: Some Cerebral Effects," *British Medical Journal*, vol. 3 (1971), pp. 67-70; and I. Oswald, S. Lewis, D. Dunleavy, V. Brezinova, and M. Briggs, "Drugs of

Dependence though Not of Abuse: Fenfluramine and Imipramine," *British Medical Journal*, vol. 3 (1971), pp. 70-73.

[64] British Medical Association Working Party Report, "Control of Amphetamine Preparations," *British Medical Journal*, vol. 4 (1968), pp. 572-73.

[65] Follows, "A Comparative Trial," pp. 236-38; H. Waal-Manning and O. Simpson, "Fenfluramine in Obese Patients on Various Antihypertensive Drugs: A Double-Blind Controlled Trial," *Lancet*, vol. 2 (1969), pp. 1392-95.

[66] H. Matthew, A. Proudfoot, R. Aitken, J. Raeburn, and N. Wright, "Nitrazepam: A Safe Hypnotic," *British Medical Journal*, vol. 3 (1969), pp. 23-25; H. Matthew, P. Roscoe, and N. Wright, "Acute Poisoning: A Comparison of Hypnotic Drugs," *Practitioner*, vol. 208 (1972), pp. 254-58.

[67] R. Mattson, "The Benzodiazepines," in *Antiepileptic Drugs*, ed. D. Woodbury, J. Penry, and R. Schmidt (New York: Raven Press, 1972), pp. 497-516.

[68] Matthew et al., "Acute Poisoning," pp. 254-58.

[69] A. J. Gardner, "Ban on Amphetamines and Barbiturates," *British Journal of Medicine*, vol. 4 (1970), pp. 801-2; H. Matthew, "Ban on Amphetamines and Barbiturates," *British Medical Journal*, vol. 4 (1970), p. 801; F. Wells, "Ban on Barbiturates?" *British Medical Journal*, vol. 4 (1970), p. 552.

[70] A. W. S. Thompson, "The Prescribing of Hypnotics, Tranquilizers and Stimulant Drugs in New Zealand: A Study of Trends over a Thirteen Year Period," Extract from the *Board of Health Report* (Wellington, New Zealand), series no. 18 (1973).

[71] U.S. Food and Drug Administration, "Legal Status of Approved Labelling for Prescription Drugs: Prescribing for Uses Unapproved by the Food and Drug Administration," *Federal Register*, vol. 37, no. 158 (1972), pp. 16,503-16,505.

[72] National Center for Health Statistics, Department of Health, Education and Welfare, *Deaths from Accidental Poisonings* (Bethesda, Md., 1972).

[73] C. Whitten, G. Gibson, M. Good, J. Goodwin, and A. Brough, "Studies in Acute Iron Poisoning I. Desferrioxamine in the Treatment of Acute Iron Poisoning: Clinical Observations, Experimental Studies, and Theoretical Considerations," *Pediatrics*, vol. 36 (1965), pp. 322-35.

[74] Ibid.; J. Crotty, "Acute Iron Poisoning in Children," *Clinical Toxicology*, vol. 4 (1971), pp. 615-19; W. Westlin, "Deferoxamine as a Chelating Agent," *Clinical Toxicology*, vol. 4 (1971), pp. 597-602.

[75] J. Robson and F. Sullivan, eds. *A Symposium on Carbenoxolone Sodium* (London: Butterworths, 1968).

[76] J. H. Thompson, "Gastrointestinal Disorders—Peptic Ulcer Disease," in *Search for New Drugs*, A. Rubin, ed., Medicinal Research Series 6 (New York: Marcel Dekker, Inc., 1972), pp. 116-200.

[77] J. Cocking and J. MacCaig, "Effect of Low Dosage of Carbenoxolone Sodium on Gastric Ulcer Healing and Acid Secretion," *Gut*, vol. 10 (1969), pp. 219-25; R. Doll, I. D. Hill, C. Hutton, and D. Underwood, "Clinical Trial of a Triterpenoid Liquorice Compound in Gastric and Duodenal Ulcer," *Lancet*, vol. 2 (1962), pp. 793-96; P. Fraser, R. Doll, M. Langman, J. Misiewicz, and H. Shawdon, "Clinical Trial of a New Carbenoxolone Analogue (BX24), Zinc Sulphate, and Vitamin A in the Treatment of Gastric Ulcer," *Gut*, vol. 13 (1972), pp. 459-62; M. Langman, "Carbenoxolone Sodium," *Gut*, vol. 9 (1968), pp. 5-6.

[78] R. Doll, M. Langman, and H. Shawdon, "Effect of Different Doses of Carbenoxolone and Different Diuretics," in *Symposium on Carbenoxolone Sodium*, ed. Robson and Sullivan, pp. 51-57.

[79] F. Avery Jones, "General Introduction," in *Symposium on Carbenoxolone Sodium*, ed. Robson and Sullivan, pp. 1-3.

[80] G. Watkinson, "Summing Up," in *Symposium on Carbenoxolone Sodium*, ed. Robson and Sullivan, pp. 245-53.

[81] Wardell, "British Usage and American Awareness of New Therapeutic Drugs," pp. 1022-34.

[82] H. E. Simmons, "Proceedings of the National Advisory Drug Committee, September 28, 1972," typescript (Washington, D. C.: Food and Drug Administration), p. 27.

[83] Wardell, "British Usage and American Awareness of New Therapeutic Drugs," pp. 1022-34; Avery Jones, "General Introduction," pp. 1-3.

[84] A. Handley, "Metoclopramide in the Prevention of Postoperative Nausea and Vomiting," *British Journal of Clinical Practice*, vol. 9 (1967), pp. 460-62; J. Traffors, A. Fisher, S. Marshall, and A. Douthwaite, "Metoclopramide (Maxolon) —A New Antiemetic," *British Journal of Clinical Practice*, vol. 9 (1967), pp. 457-60.

[85] W. James and A. Melrose, "Metoclopramide in Gastrointestinal Radiology," *Clinical Radiology*, vol. 20 (1969), pp. 57-60; A. Mitchell and R. Parkins, "Metoclopramide as an Adjunct to Small Bowel Intubation," *Gut*, vol. 10 (1969), p. 690.

[86] A. G. Johnson, "Controlled Trial of Metoclopramide in Treatment of Flatulent Dyspepsia," *British Medical Journal*, vol. 2 (1971), pp. 25-26.

[87] M. Grossman, "Gastrointestinal Hormones: Some Thoughts about Clinical Applications," *Scandinavian Journal of Gastroenterology*, vol. 7 (1972), pp. 97-104; M. E. Mason, G. Giles, and C. Clark, "Continuous Intravenous Pentagastrin as a Stimulant of Maximal Gastric Acid Secretion," *Gut*, vol. 10 (1969), pp. 34-38; Multicenter Pilot Study, "Pentagastrin as a Stimulant of Maximal Gastric Acid Response in Man," *Lancet*, vol. 1 (1967), pp. 291-95.

[88] National Academy of Sciences, *Report of the International Conference on Adverse Reactions Reporting Systems* (Washington, D. C., 1971).

NOTES TO CHAPTER VIII

[1] Wardell, "British Usage and American Awareness of New Therapeutic Drugs."

[2] Ibid., pp. 1022-34.

NOTES TO CHAPTER IX

[1] W. M. Wardell, "Deficiencies in the Acquisition, Dissemination and Interpretation of Information about New Drugs," *Drug Information Journal*, vol. 7, July/December 1973, pp. 63-66.

[2] "Cost Analysis of Selected Diseases: A Report to the Pharmaceutical Manufacturers Association" (Cambridge, Mass.: Arthur D. Little, Inc., 1967).

[3] Peltzman, *Regulation of Pharmaceutical Innovation*.

[4] World Health Organization, "Research Project for International Drug Monitoring," Report No. 5, mimeo. (Geneva, 1972).

[5] Ibid.

[6] R. Doll, "Unwanted Effects of Drugs," *British Medical Bulletin*, vol. 27 (1971), pp. 25-31; W. Inman, "Role of Drug-Reaction Monitoring in the Investigation of Thrombosis and 'The Pill,'" *British Medical Bulletin*, vol. 26 (1970), pp. 248-56; W. Inman and D. Price-Evans, "Evaluation of Spontaneous Reports of Adverse Drug Reactions," *British Medical Journal*, vol. 3 (1972), pp. 746-49; D. Mansel-Jones, "The Role of the Committee on Safety of Drugs," *British Medical Bulletin*, vol. 26 (1970), pp. 257-59.

[7] U.S. Food and Drug Administration, Advisory Committee on Obstetrics and Gynecology, *Report on the Oral Contraceptives* (Washington, D. C., 1966), and *Second Report on the Oral Contraceptives* (Washington, D. C., 1969).

[8] O. Wade, *Adverse Reactions to Drugs* (London: Medical Books, Ltd., 1970).

[9] Stolley, "Asthma Mortality," pp. 883-90.

[10] Inman and Price-Evans, "Evaluation of Spontaneous Reports," pp. 746-49.

[11] New Zealand Committee on Adverse Drug Reactions, "Three-Year Survey of Reactions, 1969-1971," *New Zealand Medical Journal*, vol. 76 (1972), pp. 100-4, and "Seventh Annual Report," *New Zealand Medical Journal*, vol. 76 (1972), pp. 357-64.

[12] World Health Organization, "Research Project, 1972."

[13] New Zealand Committee on Adverse Drug Reactions, "Three-Year Survey," pp. 100-4, and "Seventh Annual Report," pp. 357-64.

[14] S. Shapiro, D. Slone, D. Lewis, and H. Jick, "Fatal Drug Reactions among Medical Inpatients," *Journal of the American Medical Association*, vol. 216 (1971), pp. 467-72.

[15] R. Ogilvie and J. Ruedy, "Adverse Drug Reactions during Hospitalization," *Canadian Medical Association Journal*, vol. 97 (1967), pp. 1450-57.

[16] Wardell, "Introduction of New Therapeutic Drugs," pp. 773-90.

[17] Great Britain, Department of Health and Social Security, Medicines and Food Division, Committee on Safety of Medicines, *Edited and Selected Extracts from the Register of Adverse Drug Reactions* (London, 1972), covering the period January 1964 to October 1971.

[18] Simmons, Statement before the Subcommittee on Monopoly.

[19] Rustia and Shubik, "Induction of Lung Tumours," pp. 721-29.

[20] Simmons, Statement before the Subcommittee on Monopoly.

[21] *British Pharmaceutical Index.*

[22] *Monthly Index of Medical Specialties,* vol. 13, no. 9 (London: Haymarket Publishing Ltd., Medical Division, 1971).

[23] *Physicians' Desk Reference* (Oradell, N.J.: Medical Economics, Inc., 1972).

[24] Peltzman, *Regulation of Pharmaceutical Innovation*, p. 81.

[25] Great Britain, National Economic Development Office, Pharmaceuticals Working Party, Chemicals Economic Development Committee, *Focus on Pharmaceuticals* (London, 1972). This report was prepared at the invitation of the minister of health following a recommendation in the Sainsbury Report on the pharmaceutical industry and the National Health Service.

[26] Mansel-Jones, "The Role of the Committee," pp. 257-59; D. Dunlop, "The British System of Drug Regulation," unpublished paper presented at a conference on the Regulation of the Introduction of New Pharmaceuticals, sponsored by the Center for Policy Study, University of Chicago, 1972.

[27] Dunlop, "The British System of Drug Regulation," and Dunlop, "The Control of Drugs and Therapeutic Freedom," *Proceedings of the Royal Society of Medicine*, vol. 61 (1968), pp. 841-46.

[28] Great Britain, Department of Health and Social Security, Committee on Safety of Medicines, *Report for 1971* (London: Her Majesty's Stationery Office, 1972).

[29] Dunlop, "The British System of Drug Regulation."

NOTES TO CHAPTER XI

[1] Peltzman, *Regulation of Pharmaceutical Innovation*, pp. 46-48.

[2] J. M. Jadlow, "Price Competition and the Efficacy of Prescription Drugs: Conflicting Objectives?" *Nebraska Journal of Economics and Business*, vol. 11 (Autumn 1972), pp. 121-33.

[3] A. M. Schmidt, commissioner of the Food and Drug Administration, Statement before the Subcommittee on Health, Committee on Labor and Public Welfare, United States Senate, August 16, 1974; M. J. Finkel, "The Benefit/Risk Ratio of New Drug Regulation in the United States," editorial, *The Internist*, vol. 15 (1974), pp. 10-15; H. Simmons, Testimony before the Select Committee on Small Business, U.S. Senate, *Hearings on Competitive Problems in the Drug Industry*, 93rd Congress, 1st session, 1973, part 23, p. 9422.

[4] J. F. Calimlim, W. M. Wardell, L. Lasagna, A. J. Gillies, and H. T. Davis, "Effect of Naloxone on the Analgesic Activity of Methadone in a 1:10 Oral Combination," *Clinical Pharmacology and Therapeutics*, vol. 15 (1974), pp. 556-64.

NOTES TO CHAPTER XII

[1] A. Feinstein, "How Do We Measure 'Safety' and 'Efficacy'?" pp. 544-58, and "The Need for Humanized Science in Evaluating Medication," *Lancet*, vol. 2 (1972).

[2] Wardell, "Introduction of New Therapeutic Drugs," pp. 773-90.

[3] W. M. Wardell, "Control of Drug Utilization in the Context of a National Health Service: The New Zealand System," *Clinical Pharmacology and Therapeutics*, vol. 16 (1974), pp. 585-94.

[4] American Medical Association, House of Delegates, "Draft Resolutions."

[5] J. Litchfield, "Evaluation of the Safety of New Drugs by Means of Tests in Animals," *Clinical Pharmacology and Therapeutics*, vol. 3 (1962), pp. 665-72.

[6] W. M. Wardell, "Fluroxene and the Penicillin Lesson," *Anesthesiology*, vol. 38 (1973), pp. 309-12.

[7] J. C. Krantz, Jr., "Alexander Fleming and Penicillin," *Historical Medical Classics Involving New Drugs* (Baltimore: Williams and Wilkins Co., 1974), Chapter 14.

[8] A. D. Welch, "Critical Problems of Benefit versus Risk in the Development of New Drugs," paper presented at a symposium on the Development and Proper Use of New Drugs, Melbourne, November 1973, forthcoming.

[9] J. Barnes and F. Denz, "Experimental Methods Used in Determining Chronic Toxicity," *Pharmacology Review*, vol. 6 (1954), p. 191.

[10] Food and Drug Administration, Ophthalmic Advisory Committee, "Report of the Meeting, August 6-7, 1973," *Food, Drug and Cosmetic Reports*, August 13, 1973, p. 18.

[11] World Health Organization, "Research Project for International Drug Monitoring," Report No. 3, 1972.

[12] The Comptroller General of the United States, *A Report to the Congress: Assessment of the Food and Drug Administration's Handling of Reports on Adverse Reactions from the Use of Drugs* (Washington, D. C.: U.S. General Accounting Office, 1974).

[13] Wardell, "Control of Drug Utilization," pp. 585-94.

NOTES TO CHAPTER XIII

[1] C. Djerassi, "Research Impact Statements," *Science*, vol. 181 (1973), p. 115.

[2] Food and Drug Administration, *Federal Food, Drug and Cosmetic Act, as Amended, August 1972* (Washington, D. C.: Government Printing Office, 1972).

[3] The President's Science Advisory Committee, *Report of the Panel on Chemicals and Health*, NSF 73-500 (Washington, D. C.: National Science Foundation, 1973), pp. 13-15.

[4] W. H. Lyle, "Drugs for Rare Diseases," *Postgraduate Medical Journal*, vol. 50 (1974), pp. 107-8; "Drugs for Rare Diseases: Whose Responsibility?" *Lancet*, vol. 1 (1974), p. 440.

[5] Great Britain, Pharmaceuticals Working Party of the Chemicals Economic Development Committee, National Economic Development Office, "Commercially Unattractive Research," in *Focus on Pharmaceuticals* (London: Her Majesty's Stationery Office, 1972), pp. 45-47.

[6] C. G. Zubrod, "Development and Marketing of Prescription Drugs," U.S. Senate, Subcommittee on Monopoly of the Select Committee on Small Business, *Hearings on Competitive Problems in the Drug Industry,* 93rd Congress, 1st session, 1973, part 23, pp. 9672-88.

[7] Ibid.

[8] Wardell, "Fluroxene," pp. 309-12; M. Tishler, "Reflections on Drug Research and Development," mimeo., lecture given at Churchill College, Cambridge, England, 1972.

[9] C. Martin, "Phase II Evaluation of Anti-Gram-Negative Rod Antibiotics," paper presented at a symposium on Methods in Clinical Pharmacology, Phase I-II, New Orleans, 1973, forthcoming.

[10] E. A. Carr, "Clinical Pharmacology and the Human Volunteer," *Clinical Pharmacology and Therapeutics,* vol. 13 (1972), pp. 790-95.

[11] J. R. Crout, personal communication to the authors, 1974.

[12] J. Cooper, ed., *The Quality of Advice* (Washington, D. C.: Interdisciplinary Communication Associates, Inc., 1971).

[13] Zubrod, "Development and Marketing of Prescription Drugs," pp. 9672-88.

[14] Ibid.

[15] The Medicines Act (London: Her Majesty's Stationery Office, 1968).

[16] "Legal Status of Approved Labelling for Prescription Drugs: Prescribing for Uses Unapproved by the Food and Drug Administration," *Federal Register,* vol. 37, no. 158 (1972), pp. 16,503-5; J. R. Crout, Testimony at the Hearings before the Subcommittee of the Committee on Government Operations, U.S. House of Representatives, 93rd Congress, 2d session, in *Use of Advisory Committees by the Food and Drug Administration* (Washington, D. C.: Government Printing Office, 1974), p. 253; R. P. Bergen, "Prescription of Drugs Contrary to Package-Insert Recommendations," *Journal of the American Medical Association,* vol. 220 (1972), p. 1506.

[17] U.S. Congress, Senate, Subcommittee on Health, Committee on Labor and Public Welfare, *Hearings on the Quality of Health Care, Human Experimentation, I,* 93rd Congress, 1st session, February 21, 1973.

[18] "Eternal Vigilance—The Price of Liberty," editorial, *Journal of the American Medical Association,* vol. 222 (1972), pp. 1553-55; American Medical Association, House of Delegates, "Draft Resolutions."

[19] "Legal Status of Approved Labelling," pp. 16,503-5.

[20] Wardell, "Control of Drug Utilization," pp. 585-94.

[21] The Medicines Act, 1968 and 1971.

[22] Stephen L. DeFelice, *Drug Discovery: The Pending Crisis* (New York: Medcom, Inc., 1972).

[23] Food and Drug Administration, "Clinical Data on New Drugs Generated Outside the United States: Proposal to Adopt International Clinical Research Standards," *Federal Register,* vol. 38, no. 172 (September 6, 1973), pp. 24220-22.

[24] "Legal Status of Approved Labelling," pp. 16,503-5.

[25] U.S. Congress, House of Representatives, Subcommittee on Intergovernmental Relations, Committee on Government Operations, *Hearings on the Use of Advisory Committees by the Food and Drug Administration,* 93rd Congress, 2d session, 1974.

[26] C. Anello, executive secretary of the Food and Drug Administration, summary minutes of the Biometric and Epidemiological Advisory Committee, May 16, 1973.

[27] W. M. Wardell, "Assessment of the Benefits, Risks and Costs of Medical Progress," *Benefits and Risks in Medical Care* (London: Office of Health Economics, 1975).

[28] S. Gardner, acting commissioner of food and drugs, a letter to Senator Gaylord Nelson, commenting on the Pharmaceutical Manufacturers Association analysis and rebuttal of the Food and Drug Administration's testimony, July 5, 1973.

29 U.S. Congress, House, *Hearings on the Use of Advisory Committees by the Food and Drug Administration*; U.S. Congress, Senate, Health Subcommittee of the Committee on Labor and Public Welfare, *Proceedings*, August 16, 1974.

NOTES TO APPENDIX

1 D. Dunlop, "The British System of Drug Regulation," in *Regulating New Drugs*, ed. R. L. Landau (Chicago: Center for Policy Study, University of Chicago, 1973), pp. 229-37.

2 Although this and other studies have dealt with one particular sector, the introduction of new drugs, in which the losses during the 1962 amendments' first decade of operation appear to have outweighed the gains, this does not mean that the law itself is at fault; what we are seeing is the result of relatively subtle nuances in the law's interpretation and application. Nor does it mean that the law has not been well applied in all sectors; there have, on the contrary, been such obvious and important benefits as elevation of the standards of drug investigation and control of drug promotion. It would be highly desirable to have objective measures of the law's total effects, but at present there are insufficient data to allow this.

3 A. L. Cochrane, *Effectiveness and Efficiency: Random Reflections on Health Services* (London: The Nuffield Provincial Hospitals Trust, 1972).